Pocket
Prescriber

Timothy R.J. Nicholson
MBBS (London), BSc (London), MSc (Oxon),
MRCP (UK), MRCPsych (UK)
Having trained in General Medicine
at the Hammersmith Hospital, London,
he is currently training in Psychiatry
at the Maudsley Hospital, London

Editorial Advisor:
Donald R.J. Singer BMedBiol, MD, FRCP
Professor of Clinical Pharmacology, Clinical
Pharmacology Section, Leicester–Warwick
Medical Schools, University of Warwick,
Coventry, UK

Hodder Arnold

A MEMBER OF THE HODDER HEADLINE GROUP

First published in Great Britain in 2004
This second edition published in Great Britain in 2007 by
Hodder Arnold, an imprint of Hodder Education,
part of Hachette Livre UK, 38 Euston Road, London NW1 3BH

http://www.hoddereducation.com

British Library Cataloguing in Publication Data
A catalogue record for this book is available from the British Library

Library of Congress Cataloging-in-Publication Data
A catalog record for this book is available from the Library of Congress

ISBN 978 0 340 93907 9

10

Commissioning Editor: Philip Shaw
Project Editor: Heather Fyfe
Production Controller: Karen Tate
Cover Design: Laura Degrasse

Typeset in 8/10 pt Sabon by Charon Tec Ltd (A Macmillan Company), Chennai, India
www.charontec.com
Printed and bound in Spain

What do you think about this book? Or any other Arnold title?
Please visit our website at www.hoddereducation.com

CONTENTS

Algorithms

ACKNOWLEDGEMENTS

This book is dedicated to my family and friends as well as all the inspirational teachers I have been lucky enough to learn from over the years, in particular John Youle, Katie Blackman, Jerry Kirk, Carol Black, Huw Beynon, Martin Rossor, Michael Trimble and Maria Ron.

Particular thanks for their help and time to Anand and Subbu, Houman Ashrafian, Nick Bateman, Gurpreet Chana, Roger Cross, Jonny Crowston, Chris Denton, Emma Derritt-Smith, Samantha Dickinson, Paul Dilworth, Tim Doulton, Michael Duick, Phil Dyer, Nick Eynon-Lewis, Fahad Farooqi, Catherine Farrow, Roger Fernandes, Arosha Fernando, Denise Forth, Jack Galliford, Thomas Galliford, Hamid Ghodse, Natasha Gilani, Peter Hargreaves, Nicholas Hirsch, Rick Holliman, Nick Jackson, Sudhesh Kumar, Graham MacGregor, Mel Mahadevan, Omar Malik, Chung Man Wan, Jane Marshall, Narbeh Melikian, Alli Morton, Neil Muchatuta, Dev Mukerjee, Gideon Paul, Tejal Patel, Rahul Patel, Rakita Patel, Annabel Price, Muriel Shannon, Amar Sharif, Jennifer Sharp, Bran Sivakumar, Sian Stanley, Richard Stratton, Henry Squire, Sheena Thomas, Mike Travis, Aaron Vallance and Jim Wade.

Special thanks to Helen Galley.

The information in this book has been collated from many sources, including manufacturer's information sheets ('SPCs' – summary of product characteristics sheets), the British National Formulary (BNF), national and international guidelines, as well as numerous pharmacology and general medical books, journals and papers. Where information is not consistent between these sources that from the SPCs has generally been taken as definitive.

FOREWORD

Contemporary medical practice necessitates a broad knowledge of drug treatments, which are constantly being updated and modified. I am delighted to write the foreword for this volume which, in the principle of the very best travel guides, is small but packed with essential and easily accessible information. Of all the subjects that are in the medical curriculum, pharmacology can sometimes seem especially abstract and theoretical. A quick flick through the pages of this book that are relevant to one's own speciality is an immediate reminder of the importance of understanding the ways in which the drugs that we routinely prescribe are handled. The clear identification of hazardous side-effects and potential interactions is especially welcome. Finally, the section providing current information and management guidelines for commonly encountered medical emergencies is both clear and comprehensive.

Safe use of the modern therapeutic armamentarium is a daunting task for junior doctors and medical students. Although there has been a large growth in electronic resources and some excellent on-line textbooks have been produced, there remains a critical need for small reference texts that can be carried at all times and used to check drug doses or potential interactions at the point of prescription. The simple precaution of checking facts in any unfamiliar prescribing situation is likely to prevent mistakes, and exemplifies current emphasis on safe-practice and clinical risk management.

I believe that even the most senior specialist could learn something from this book's pages and that a comprehensive up-to-date volume such as this is an essential part of any junior doctor's tool kit, and will prove useful far beyond its target audience.

Professor Dame Carol M. Black DBE
President of the Royal College of Physicians

HOW TO USE THIS BOOK

The aim of this pocket book is to provide the reference information needed for the majority of prescriptions made by a junior doctor, along with practical prescribing advice. By its nature it will omit much detail, which can of course be found in other sources. The information is highly keyed and condensed, but once you are familiar with the format, it should be quick to use, save you much time, and enable more frequent checks and subsequently safer prescribing.

IMPORTANT INFORMATION

This book is not comprehensive. Not all features of each drug (in particular, side effects and interactions) are mentioned. Only important and 'need-to-know' information is included.

If you need further information about specific drugs, please consult other sources, such as manufacturers' information sheets, the *British National Formulary* (BNF), your pharmacy, and your clinical colleagues.

It must also be noted that this book is based on current prescribing practice in the UK so drug nomenclature, formulations, doses and guidelines for use reflect this. Readers in countries outside the UK should ensure that information in the book is used in the context of their national advice on medical practice and prescribing.

Any errors noted and comments on how to improve this book will be received gratefully. Please write with your comments or suggestions to Dr Timothy R.J. Nicholson, Pocket Prescriber, c/o Hodder Arnold, Health Sciences, 338 Euston Road, London NW1 3BH, UK or email pocketprescriber@hodder.co.uk.

STANDARD LAYOUT OF DRUGS

DRUG/TRADE NAME

Class/action: More information is given for generic forms, especially for the original and most commonly used drug(s) of each class.

Use: use^x (correlating to dose as below).

CI: contraindications; **L** (liver failure), **R** (renal failure), **H** (heart failure), **P** (pregnancy), **B** (breastfeeding). *Allergy to active drug, or any excipients (other substances in the preparation) assumed too obvious to mention.*

Caution: **L** (liver failure), **R** (renal failure), **H** (heart failure), **P** (pregnancy), **B** (breastfeeding), **E** (elderly patients).

SE: side effects; listed in order of frequency encountered. Common/ important side effects set in **bold**.

Warn: information to give to patients before starting drug.

Monitor: parameters that need to be monitored during treatment.

Interactions: included only if very common or potentially serious; ↑/↓**P450** (induces/inhibits cytochrome P450 metabolism), **W+** (increases effect of warfarin), **W−** (decreases effect of warfarin).

Dose: dose^x (for Use^x as above). *NB Doses are for adults only.*

Important points highlighted at end of drug entry.

Use/dose^{NICE}: National Institute of Health and Clinical Excellence guidelines exist for the drug (basics often in BNF – see www.nice.org.uk for full details).

Dose$^{BNF/SPC}$: dose regimen complicated; please refer to BNF and/or SPC (Summary of Product Characteristic sheet; manufacturer's information sheet enclosed with drug packaging – can also be viewed at or downloaded from www.emc.medicines.org.uk).

Asterisks (*) and **daggers** (†) denote links between information within local text.

Only relevant sections are included for each drug.

Trade names (in OUTLINE font) are given only if found regularly on drug charts or if non-proprietary (generic, non-trade-name) drug does not exist yet.

KEY

- ☠ Potential dangers highlighted with skull and cross-bones
- ▼ New drug or new indication under intense surveillance by Committee on Safety of Medicines (CSM): *important to report all suspected drug reactions via Yellow Card scheme* (accurate as going to press: from June 2006 CSM list)
- ☺ *Good for:* reasons to give a certain drug when choice exists
- ☻ *Bad for:* reasons to not give a certain drug when choice exists
- ⇒ Causes/goes to
- ∴ Therefore
- Δ Change/disturbance
- Ψ Psychiatric
- ↑ Increase/high
- ↓ Decrease/low

↑/↓ electrolytes refers to serum levels, unless stated otherwise.

DOSES

od	once daily	nocte	at night
bd	twice daily	mane	in the morning
tds	three times daily	prn	as required
qds	four times daily	stat	at once

ROUTES

im	intramuscular	po	oral
inh	inhaled	pr	rectal
iv	intravenous	sc	subcutaneous
ivi	intravenous infusion	top	topical
neb	via nebuliser		

Routes are presumed po, unless stated otherwise.

ABBREVIATIONS

AAC	antibiotic-associated colitis
Ab	antibody
ACE-i	ACE inhibitor
ACh	acetylcholine
ACS	acute coronary syndrome
AF	atrial fibrillation
Ag	antigen
ALL	acute lymphoblastic leukaemia
AMI	acute myocardial infarction
AMTS	abbreviated mental test score (same as MTS)
ANA	anti-nuclear antigens
5-ASA	5-aminosalicylic acid
AV	arteriovenous
AVM	arteriovenous malformation
AVN	atrioventricular node
AZT	zidovudine
ARB(s)	angiotensin receptor blocker(s)
ARDS	adult respiratory distress syndrome
ARF	acute renal failure
AS	aortic stenosis
ASAP	as soon as possible
BBB	bundle branch block
BCSH	British Committee for Standards in Haematology
BCT	broad complex tachycardia
BF	blood flow
BG	serum blood glucose; *see also CBG*
BHS	British Hypertension Society
BIH	benign intracranial hypertension
BM	bone marrow (NB: BM is often used, confusingly, to signify finger-prick glucose; CBG (capillary blood glucose) is used for this purpose in this book)
BMI	body mass index = weight (kg)/height (m)^2
BP	blood pressure
BPH	benign prostatic hypertrophy
BTS	British Thoracic Society
Bx	biopsy
C	constipation
Ca	cancer (NB: calcium is abbreviated to Ca^{2+})
CAH	congenital adrenal hyperplasia

CBF	cerebral blood flow
CBG	capillary blood glucose (finger-prick testing) (NB: BM is often used to denote this, but this is confusing and less accurate and thus not used in this book)
CCF	congestive cardiac failure
cf	compared with
CI	contraindicated
CK	creatine kinase
CLL	chronic lymphocytic leukaemia
CML	chronic myelogenous leukaemia
CMV	cytomegalovirus
CNS	central nervous system
CO	cardiac output
COPD	chronic obstructive pulmonary disease
COX	cyclo-oxygenase
CPR	cardiopulmonary resuscitation
CRF	chronic renal failure
CSF	cerebrospinal fluid
CSM	Committee on Safety of Medicines
CVA	cerebrovascular accident
CVP	central venous pressure
CXR	chest X-ray
D	diarrhoea
$D_{1/2/3 \ldots}$	dopamine receptor subtype 1/2/3 ...
DA	dopamine
DCT	distal convoluted tubule
dfx	defects
DI	diabetes insipidus
DIGAMI	glucose, insulin and potassium intravenous infusion used in acute myocardial infarction
DKA	diabetic ketoacidosis
DM	diabetes mellitus
DMARD	disease-modifying anti-rheumatoid arthritis drug
dt	due to
D&V	diarrhoea and vomiting
Dx	diagnosis
EBV	Epstein–Barr virus
ECG	electrocardiogram
ECT	electroconvulsive therapy
e'lyte	electrolyte
ENT	ear, nose and throat

EØ	eosinophils
EPSE	extrapyramidal side effects
ERC	European Resuscitation Council
ESC	European Society of Cardiology
ESR	erythrocyte sedimentation rate
exac	exacerbates
FBC	full blood count
Fe	iron
FFP	fresh frozen plasma
FiO$_2$	inspired O$_2$ concentration
FMF	Familial Mediterranean Fever
fx	effects
GABA	gamma aminobutyric acid
GBS	Guillain–Barré syndrome
GCS	Glasgow coma scale
GI	gastrointestinal
GIK	glucose, insulin and K$^+$ infusion
G6PD	glucose-6-phosphate dehydrogenase
GU	genitourinary
h	hour(s)
HB	heart block
Hct	haematocrit
HDL	high density lipoprotein
HF	heart failure
HIV	human immunodeficiency virus
HMG-CoA	3-hydroxy-3-methyl-glutaryl coenzyme A
H(O)CM	hypertrophic (obstructive) cardiomyopathy
HONK	hyperosmolar non-ketotic state
hrly	hourly
HSV	herpes simplex virus
5-HT	5-hydroxytryptamine (= serotonin)
HTN	hypertension
HUS	haemolytic uraemic syndrome
Hx	history
IBD	inflammatory bowel disease
IBS	irritable bowel syndrome
ICP	intracranial pressure
ICU	intensive care unit
IHD	ischaemic heart disease
inc	including
im	intramuscular

IOP	intraocular pressure
ITP	immune/idiopathic thrombocytopoenic purpura
ITU	intensive therapy unit
iv	intravenous
ivi	intravenous infusion
Ix	investigation
IVDU	intravenous drug user
K^+	potassium (serum levels unless stated otherwise)
LA	long-acting
LBBB	left bundle branch block
LDL	low density lipoprotein
LF	liver failure
LFTs	liver function tests
LØ	lymphocytes
LP	lumbar puncture
LVF	left ventricular failure
mane	in morning
MAOI	monoamine oxidase inhibitor
MAP	mean arterial pressure
metab	metabolised
MG	myasthenia gravis
MHRA	Medicines and Healthcare Products Regulatory Authority (UK)
MI	myocardial infarction
MMF	mycophenolate mofetil
MMSE	mini mental state examination (scored out of 30*)
MØ	macrophages
MR	modified-release (drug preparation)
MRSA	methicillin-resistant *Staphylococcus aureus*
MS	multiple sclerosis
MTS	(abbreviated) mental test score (scored out of 10*)
Mx	management
N	nausea
Na^+	sodium (serum levels unless stated otherwise)
NA	noradrenaline (norepinephrine)
NBM	nil by mouth
NCT	narrow complex tachycardia
NGT	nasogastric tube
NIV	non-invasive ventilation
NMJ	neuromuscular junction
NMS	neuroleptic malignant syndrome

NØ	neutrophils
NPIS	National Poisons Information Service
NSAID	nonsteroidal anti-inflammatory drug
NSTEMI	non-ST elevation myocardial infarction
N&V	nausea and vomiting
OCD	obsessive compulsive disorder
OCP	oral contraceptive pill
OD	overdose (*NB: od = once daily!*)
PAN	polyarteritis nodosa
PBC	primary biliary cirrhosis
PCOS	polycystic ovary syndrome
PCI	percutaneous coronary intervention (now preferred term for percutaneous transluminal coronary angioplasty (PTCA), which is a subtype of PCI)
PCP	*Pneumocystis carinii* pneumonia
PDA	patent ductus arteriosus
PE	pulmonary embolism
PEA	pulseless electrical activity
PEG	percutaneous endoscopic gastrostomy
PG(*x*)	prostaglandin (receptor subtype *x*)
phaeo	phaeochromocytoma
PHx	past history (of)
PID	pelvic inflammatory disease
PMR	polymyalgia rheumatica
PO_4	phosphate (serum levels, unless stated otherwise)
po	by mouth
PPI	proton pump inhibitor
prep(s)	preparation(s)
prn	as required
Pt	platelet(s)
PT	prothrombin time
PTH	parathyroid hormone
PU	peptic ulcer
PUO	pyrexia of unknown origin
PVD	peripheral vascular disease
p'way(s)	pathway(s)
Px	prophylaxis
QT(c)	QT interval (corrected for rate)
RA	rheumatoid arthritis
RAS	renal artery stenosis
RBF	renal blood flow

RF	renal failure
RR	respiratory rate
RVF	right ventricular failure
Rx	treatment
SAH	subarachnoid haemorrhage
SAN	sinoatrial node
SE(s)	side effect(s)
sec(s)	second(s)
SIADH	syndrome of inappropriate antidiuretic hormone
SJS	Stevens–Johnson syndrome
sl	sublingual
SLE	systemic lupus erythematosus
SOA	swelling of ankles
SOB (OE)	shortness of breath (on exertion)
SPC	summary of product characteristic sheet (see page x)
spp	species
SR	slow/sustained release (drug preparation)
SSRI	selective serotonin reuptake inhibitor
SSS	sick sinus syndrome
STEMI	ST elevation myocardial infarction
SVT	supraventricular tachycardia
supp	suppository
T_3	triiodothyronine/liothyronine
T_4	thyroxine ($\uparrow/\downarrow T_4$ = hyper/hypothyroid)
$t_{1/2}$	half-life
TCA	tricyclic antidepressant
TE	thromboembolism
TEDS	thromboembolism deterrent stockings
TEN	toxic epidermal necrolysis
TFTs	thyroid function tests
TG	triglyceride
TNF	tumour necrosis factor
TPMT	thiopurine methyltransferase
TPR	total peripheral resistance
TTP	thrombotic thrombocytopoenic purpura
UA(P)	unstable angina (pectoris)
UC	ulcerative colitis
U&Es	urea and electrolytes
URTI	upper respiratory tract infection
UTI	urinary tract infection
UV	ultraviolet

V	vomiting
VE(s)	ventricular ectopic(s)
VF	ventricular fibrillation
vit	vitamin
VLDL	very low density lipoprotein
VT	ventricular tachycardia
VZV	varicella zoster virus (chickenpox/shingles)
w	with
WCC	white cell count
WE	Wernicke's encephalopathy
w/in	within
wk	week
w/o	without
WPW	Wolf–Parkinson–White syndrome
Wt	weight
xs	excess
ZE	Zollinger–Ellison syndrome

Common/useful drugs

ABCIXIMAB/REOPRO

Antiplatelet agent – monoclonal Ab against platelet glycoprotein IIb/IIIa receptor (involved in Pt aggregation).

Use: Px of ischaemic complications of PCI and Px of MI in unstable angina unresponsive to conventional Rx awaiting PCI[NICE] (see p. 198).

CI: Active internal bleeding. CVA w/in 2 years. Intracranial neoplasm, aneurysm or AVM. Major surgery, intracranial/intraspinal surgery or trauma w/in 2 months. Hypertensive retinopathy, vasculitis, ↓Pt, haemorrhagic diathesis, severe ↑BP. **L** (if severe)/ **R** (if requiring haemodialysis)/**B**.

Caution: drugs that ↑bleeding risk, P.

SE: bleeding*/↓Pt*, N&V, ↓BP, ↓HR, pain (chest, back or pleuritic), headache, fever. Rarely, hypersensitivity, tamponade, ARDS.

Monitor: FBC* (baseline plus 2–4 h, 12 h and 24 h after giving) and clotting (baseline at least).

Dose: 250 µg/kg iv over 1 min, then 0.125 µg/kg/min (max 10 µg/min) ivi. Needs concurrent heparin. See BNF/product literature for dose timing.

Specialist use only: get senior advice or contact on-call cardiology.

ACAMPROSATE/CAMPRAL EC

Modifies GABA transmission ⇒ ↓pleasurable fx of alcohol ∴ ↓s craving and relapse rate.

Use: maintaining alcohol abstinence.

CI: **L** (only if severe), **R/P/B**.

SE: GI upset, rash, Δ libido.

Dose: 666 mg tds po if age 18–65 years (avoid outside this age range) and >60 kg (if <60 kg give 666 mg mane then 333 mg noon and nocte). *Start ASAP after alcohol stopped. Usually give for 1 yr.*

ACETYLCYSTEINE/PARVOLEX

Precursor of glutathione, which detoxifies metabolites of paracetamol.

Use: paracetamol OD.

Caution: asthma*.

SE: allergy: rash, bronchospasm*, anaphylaxis (esp if ivi too quick**).
Dose: initially 150 mg/kg in 200 ml 5% glucose as ivi over 15 min, then 50 mg/kg in 500 ml over 4 h, then 100 mg/kg in 1 litre over 16 h. NB: use max weight of 110 kg for dose calculation, even if patient weighs more. Ensure not given too quickly**.
See pp. 211–14 for Mx of paracetamol OD and treatment line graph.

ACICLOVIR (previously **ACYCLOVIR**)
Antiviral. Inhibits DNA polymerase *only in infected cells*: needs activation by viral thymidine kinase (produced by herpes spp).
Use: *iv*: severe HSV or VZV infections, e.g. meningitis, encephalitis and in immunocompromised patients (esp HIV – also used for Px); *po/top*: mucous membrane, genital, eye infections.
Caution: dehydration*, R/P/B.
SE: at ↑doses: **ARF, encephalopathy** (esp if dehydrated*). Also **hypersensitivity**, GI upset, blood disorders, skin reactions, headache, many non-specific neurological symptoms. Rarely Ψ reactions and hepatotoxicity.
Interactions: levels ↑d by probenecid.
Dose: 5 mg/kg tds ivi over 1 h (10 mg/kg if HSV encephalitis or VZV in immunocompromised patients); po/top^SPC/BNF.
☠ ivi leaks ⇒ severe local inflammation/ulceration. ☠

ACTIVATED CHARCOAL see Charcoal

ACTRAPID Short-acting soluble insulin; see p. 166 for use.

ADENOSINE
Purine nucleoside. Slows AVN conduction, dilates coronary arteries; acts on its own specific receptors.
Use: Rx of paroxysmal SVT (esp if accessory p'ways e.g. WPW) and Dx of SVT (NCT or BCT; ↓s rate to reveal underlying rhythm).

CI: ☠ asthma* (consider verapamil instead). ☠ 2nd-/3rd-degree AV block or sick sinus syndrome (if either w/o pacemaker).
Caution: heart transplant (↓dose), AF/atrial flutter (↑s accessory pathway conduction), ↑QTc, COPD*.
SE: bronchospasm*, ↓BP. Rarely, ↓HR/asystole and arrhythmias (mostly transient).
Warn: can ⇒ transient unpleasant feelings: facial flushing, dyspnoea, choking feeling, nausea, chest pain and light-headedness.
Interactions: fx ↑by **dipyridamole**: ↓initial adenosine dose to 0.5–1 mg and watch for ↑bleeding (*anti-Pt fx of dipyridamole also ↑d by adenosine*). fx ↓d by **theophyllines** and caffeine.
Dose: 3–6 mg iv over 2 secs; double dose and repeat every 1–2 min until response or significant AV block (max 12 mg/dose). NB: attach cardiac monitor and give via central (or large peripheral) vein, then flush.

$t_{1/2}$ <10 s: often needs readministration (esp if given for Rx cf Dx).

ADRENALINE (im/iv)

Sympathomimetic: powerful stimulation of α (vasoconstriction), β_1 (↑HR, ↑contractility) and β_2 (vasodilation, bronchodilation, uterine relaxation).
Use: CPR and anaphylaxis (see algorithms on inside and outside front cover, respectively). Rarely for other causes of bronchospasm or shock (e.g. 2° to spinal/ epidural anaesthesia).
Caution: cerebrovascular* and heart disease (esp arrhythmias and HTN), DM, ↑T4, glaucoma (angle closure), labour (esp 2nd stage). H/E.
SE: ↑HR, ↑BP, anxiety, sweats, tremor, headache, peripheral vasoconstriction, arrhythmias, pulmonary oedema (at ↑doses), N&V, weakness, dizziness, Ψ disturbance, hyperglycaemia, urinary retention (esp if ↑prostate). Rarely CVA* (2° to HTN: monitor BP).
Interactions: fx ↑d by TCAs, ergotamine and oxytocin. Risk of: 1. ↑↑BP and ↓HR with β-blockers; 2. arrhythmias with digoxin, quinidine and volatile liquid anaesthetics (e.g. halothane).

Dose: CPR: 1 mg **iv** = 10 ml of 1 in **10 000** (100 µg/ml) then flush with ≥20 ml saline. *If no or delayed iv access, try intra-osseous route and, if this is not possible, give 2–3 mg via endotracheal tube diluted to 10 ml with sterile water.* Repeat as per ALS algorithm (see front cover). **Anaphylaxis**: 0.5 mg **im** (or sc) = 0.5 ml of 1 in **1000** (1 mg/ml); repeat after 5 min if no response. (If cardiac arrest seems imminent or concerns over im absorption, give 0.5 mg **iv** *slowly* = 5 ml of 1 in **10 000** (100 µg/ml) at 1 ml/min until response – get senior help first if possible as iv route ⇒ ↑risk of arrhythmias.) ☠Do not confuse 1 in 1000 (im) with 1:10 000 (iv) solutions. ☠

ADVIL see Ibuprofen

AGGRASTAT see Tirofiban; IIb/IIIa inhibitor (anti-Pt drug) for IHD.

ALENDRONATE (ALENDRONIC ACID)/FOSAMAX
Bisphosphonate: ↓s osteoclastic bone resorption
Use: osteoporosis Rx and Px (esp if on corticosteroids).
CI: delayed GI emptying (esp achalasia and oesophageal stricture/other abnormalities), ↓Ca^{2+}, unable to sit/stand upright ≥30 min, **P/B**.
Caution: upper GI disorders (inc gastritis/PU). **R**.
SE: oesophageal reactions*, GI upset/distension, ↓Ca^{2+}, ↓PO_4^{2-} (transient), PU, hypersensitivity (esp skin reactions).
Warn: take with full glass of water on an empty stomach ≥30 min before, and stay upright until, breakfast*. Stop tablets and seek medical attention if symptoms of oesophageal irritation develop.
Dose: 5–10 mg mane[SPC/BNF] (if 10 mg od, can give as once-weekly 70-mg tablet *if for post menopausal osteoporosis*). Take on empty stomach before other medications.

ALFACALCIDOL
1-α-hydroxycholecalciferol: partially activated vitamin D (1α hydroxy group normally added by kidney), but still requires hepatic (25)-hydroxylation for full activation.
Use: severe vitamin D deficiency, esp 2° to CRF.
CI/SE: ↑Ca^{2+}: monitor levels, watch for symptoms (esp N&V).

Interactions: fx may be ↓d by barbiturates and anticonvulsants.
Dose: 0.25–1 μg od po.

ALLOPURINOL

Xanthine oxidase inhibitor: ↓s uric acid synthesis.
Use: Px of **gout**, renal stones (urate or Ca^{2+} oxalate) and other ↑urate states (esp 2° to chemotherapy).
CI: acute gout: can worsen – do not start drug during attack (but do not stop drug if acute attack occurs during Rx).
Caution: R (↓dose), L (↓dose and monitor LFTs), P/B.
SE: GI upset, ☠**severe skin reactions**☠ (*stop drug if rash develops and allopurinol is implicated* – can reintroduce cautiously if mild reaction and no recurrence). Rarely, neuropathy (and many non-specific neurological symptoms), blood disorders, RF, hepatotoxicity.
Warn: report rashes, maintain good hydration.
Interactions: ↑s fx/toxicity of **azathioprine** (and possibly other cytotoxics, esp ciclosporin), chlorpropamide and theophyllines. Level ↓d by salicylates and probenecid, ↑rash with ampicillin and amoxicillin. **W+**.
Dose: initially 100 mg od po (↑ if required to max of 900 mg/day in divided doses of up to 300 mg) after food.

Initial Rx can ↑gout: give colchicine or NSAID (e.g. indometacin or diclofenac – *not aspirin*) Px until ≥1 month after urate normalised.

ALPHAGAN see Brimonidine; α-agonist eye drops for glaucoma

ALTEPLASE ((**R**)ecombinant) **T**issue-type **P**lasminogen **A**ctivator, rt-PA, TPA). Recombinant fibrinolytic.
Use: acute **MI**, acute massive **PE** (with haemodynamic instability). Acute ischaemic CVA w/in 3 h of onset (specialist use only).
CI/Caution/SE: See pp. 177–80 for use in MI (for use in PE/CVA, see SPC).

Dose: MI: total dose of 100 mg – regimen depends on time since onset of pain: *0–6 h*: 15 mg iv bolus, then 50 mg ivi over 30 min, then 35 mg ivi over 60 min; *6–12 h*: 10 mg iv bolus, then 50 mg ivi over 60 min, then four further 10 mg ivis, each over 30 min.
PE: 10 mg iv over 1–2 min then 90 mg ivi over 2 h.

☠️↓doses if patient <65 kg; see SPC. ☠️ If MI concurrent unfractionated iv heparin needed for ⩾24 h; see p. 179. Heparin also needed if giving for PE; see SPC.

ALUMINIUM HYDROXIDE

Antacid, PO_4 -binding agent (↓s GI absorption).
Use: dyspepsia, ↑PO_4 (which can ↑risk of bone disease; esp good if secondary to RF, when ↑Ca^{2+} can occur dt ↑PTH, as other PO_4 binders often contain Ca^{2+}).
CI: ↓PO_4, porphyria.
SE: constipation*. Aluminium can accumulate in RF (esp if dialysis) ⇒ ↑risk of encephalopathy, dementia, osteomalacia.
Interactions: can ↓absorption of oral antibiotics (e.g. tetracyclines).
Dose: 1–2 (500 mg) tablets or 5–10 ml of 4% suspension prn (qds often sufficient). ↑doses to individual requirements, esp if for ↑PO_4. Also available as 475 mg capsules as Alucaps (contains ↓Na^+).

Most effective taken with meals and at bedtime. Consider laxative Px*.

AMFEBUTAMONE see Buproprion; aid to smoking cessation.

AMILORIDE

K^+-sparing diuretic (weak): inhibits DCT Na^+ reabsorption and K^+ excretion.
Use: oedema (2° to HF, cirrhosis or ↑aldosterone), HTN (esp in conjunction with ↑K^+-wasting diuretics as combination preparations; see Co-amilofruse and Co-amilozide).
CI: ↑K^+, **R**
Caution: DM (as risk of RF; monitor U&E), ↑risk of acidosis, P/B/E.

SE: ↑K^+, **GI upset**, headache, dry mouth, ↓BP (esp postural), ↓Na^+, rash, confusion. Rarely encephalopathy, hepatic/renal dysfunction.

Interactions: ↑s lithium levels. Can ↑nephrotoxicity of NSAIDs.

Dose: 2.5–20 mg od (or divide into bd doses).

☠Beware if on other drugs that ↑K^+, e.g. spironolactone, triamterene, ACE-i, ARBs and ciclosporin. Do not give oral K^+ supplements inc dietary salt tablets. ☠

AMINOPHYLLINE

Methylxanthine bronchodilator: as theophylline but ↑H_2O solubility (is mixed w ethylenediamine) and ↓hypersensitivity.

Use/CI/Caution/SE/Monitor/Interactions: see Theophylline; also available iv for use in acute severe bronchospasm; see p. 201.

☠NB: has many important interactions (dose adjustment may be needed) and can ⇒ arrhythmias (use cardiac monitor if giving iv). ☠

Dose: po: MR preparation (Phyllocontin Continus) ⇒ ↓SEs, has different doses at 225–450 mg bd
(or 350–700 mg bd if Forte tablets – for smokers and others with short $t_{1/2}$). *If on a particular brand, ensure this is prescribed as they have different pharmacokinetics.*

iv: load* with 5 mg/kg (usually = 250–500 mg) over ⩾20 min, then 0.5 mg/kg/h ivi, then adjusted to keep plasma levels at 10–20 mg/l (= 55–110 μmol/l). If possible contact pharmacy for dosing advice to consider interactions, obesity and liver/heart function.

☠If already taking maintenance po aminophylline/theophylline, omit loading dose* and check levels ASAP to guide dosing. ☠

AMIODARONE

Class III antiarrhythmic: ↑s refractory period of conducting system; useful as has ↓negative inotropic fx than other drugs and can give when others ineffective/CI.

Use: tachyarrhythmias: esp paroxysmal SVT, AF, atrial flutter, nodal tachycardias, VT and VF. Also in CPR/peri-arrest arrhythmias.

CI: ↓HR (sinus), sinoatrial HB, SAN disease or severe conduction disturbance w/o pacemaker, Hx of thyroid disease/iodine sensitivity, **P/B**.

Caution: porphyria, ↓K$^+$ (↑risk of torsades), **L/R/H/E**.

SE: *Acute:* N&V (dose-dependent), ↓**HR/BP**. *Chronic:* rarely but seriously ↑**or** ↓**T$_4$, interstitial lung disease** (e.g. fibrosis, *but reversible if caught early*), **hepatotoxicity, conduction disturbances** (esp ↓HR). *Common:* **malaise, fatigue,** photosensitive skin (rarely 'grey-slate'), corneal deposits ± 'night glare' (reversible). *Less commonly:* optic neuritis (rare but can ↓vision), peripheral neuropathy, blood disorders, hypersensitivity.

Monitor: TFTs and LFTs (baseline then 6-monthly). Also baseline K$^+$ and CXR (watch for ↑SOB/alveolitis).

Warn: avoid sunlight/use sunscreen (inc several months after stopping).

Interactions: ↑s fx of phenytoin and digoxin. Other class III and many class Ia antiarrhythmics, antipsychotics, TCAs, lithium, erythromycin, co trimoxazole, antimalarials, nelfinavir, ritonavir ⇒ ↑risk of ventricular arrhythmias. Verapamil, diltiazem and β-blockers ⇒ ↑risk of ↓HR and HB **W+**.

Dose: **po:** load with 200 mg tds in 1st wk, 200 mg bd in 2nd wk, then (usually od) maintenance dose according to response (long t$_{1/2}$: months before steady plasma concentration); **iv:** (extreme emergencies only) 150–300 mg in 10–20 ml 5% glucose over ≥3 min (do not repeat for ≥15 min); **ivi:** 5 mg/kg over 20–120 min (max 1.2 g/day). *For use in cardiac arrest see ALS algorithm and for use in acute tachycardias, see algorithms in the cover flaps of this book.*

☠ iv doses: give via central line (if no time for insertion, give via largest Venflon possible) with ECG monitoring. Avoid giving if severe respiratory failure or ↓BP (unless caused by arrhythmia) as can worsen. Avoid iv boluses if CCF/cardiomyopathy. ☠

AMITRIPTYLINE

Tricyclic antidepressant: blocks reuptake of NA (and 5-HT).

Use: depression[1] (esp if sedation beneficial), neuropathic pain[2].

CI: recent MI (w/in 3 months), arrhythmias (esp HB), mania, **L** (if severe).

Caution: cardiac/thyroid disease, epilepsy*, glaucoma (angle closure), ↑prostate, phaeo, porphyria, anaesthesia. Also Hx of mania, psychosis or urinary retention, **H/P/B/E**.

SE: antimuscarinic fx (see p. 191), **cardiac fx** (arrhythmias, HB, ↑HR, postural ↓BP, dizziness, syncope: **dangerous in OD**), ↑**Wt, sedation**** (often ⇒ 'hangover'), seizures*, movement disorders. Rarely mania, fever, blood disorders, hypersensitivity, ΔLFTs, ↓Na^+ (esp in elderly), neuroleptic malignant syndrome.

Warn: may impair driving**.

Interactions: ☠**MAOIs** ⇒ HTN and CNS excitation. ☠ Levels ↑d by SSRIs, phenothiazines and cimetidine. ↑Risk of arrhythmias with **amiodarone, pimpozide** (is CI), thioridazine and some class I antiarrhythmics. ↑risk of paralytic ileus with antimuscarinics. ↑s sedative fx of alcohol. ↑CNS toxicity with **sibutramine** (is CI).

Dose: initially 75 mg (30–75 mg in elderly) nocte or in divided doses (↑if required to max 200 mg/day)[1].

AMLODIPINE/ISTIN

Ca^{2+} channel blocker (dihydropyridine): as nifedipine, but ⇒ no ↓contractility or ↑HF.

Use: HTN, angina (esp 'Prinzmetal's' = coronary vasospasm).

CI: ACS, cardiogenic shock, significant aortic stenosis, **P/B**.

Caution: L.

SE/Interactions: as nifedipine but ↑ankle swelling and possibly ↓vasodilator fx (headache, flushing and dizziness).

Dose: initially 5 mg od po (↑if required to 10 mg).

AMOXICILLIN

Broad-spectrum penicillin; good GI absorption (can give po and iv).

Use: mild pneumonias[1] (esp community-acquired), UTI, listeria meningitis, endocarditis Px and many ENT/dental/other infections. *Often used with clavulanic acid as co-amoxiclav.*

CI/Caution/SE/Interactions: see Ampicillin.

Dose: 500–1000 mg tds po/iv[1]; for other severe infections see SPC/BNF (mild/moderate infections usually 250–500 mg tds po).

AMPICILLIN

Broad-spectrum penicillin for iv use: has ↓GI absorption cf amoxicillin, which is preferred po.

Use: Meningitis (esp *Listeria*; see p. 147)[1], Px preoperative or for endocarditis during invasive procedures if valve lesions/prostheses, respiratory tract/ENT infections (esp community-acquired pneumonia dt *Haemophilus influenzae* or *Streptococcus pneumoniae*), UTIs (not for blind Rx, as *Escherichia coli* often resistant).

CI: penicillin hypersensitivity (NB: cross-reactivity with cefalosporins possible).

Caution: EBV/CMV infections, ALL, CLL (all ↑risk of rash), R (if severe ↓dose).

SE: rash* (erythematous, maculopapular: often does not reflect true allergy), **N&V&D** (rarely AAC), **hypersensitivity**, CNS/blood disorders.

Interactions: levels ↑ by probenecid. ↑ risk of rash with allopurinol. Can ↓ fx of OCP (warn patient) and ↑ levels of methotrexate.

Dose: 2 g 4-hourly ivi[1]; most other indications 0.25–1 g qds po/im/iv[SPC/BNF].

ANTABUSE see Disulfiram; adjunct to alcohol withdrawal.

APRACLONIDINE/IOPIDINE

Topical (ocular) α_2 agonist: ↓s aqueous humour production.

Use: glaucoma: short-term Rx of severe cases.

CI: cardiovascular disease (severe or uncontrolled – inc Hx of).

Caution: IHD, vasovagal attacks, cerebrovascular disease, depression, R/H/P/B.

SE: dry mouth, taste Δ, local pruritus/discomfort (oedema), headache, asthenia, dry nose. NB: systemic fx can occur and **Interactions** theoretically possible (see Clonidine).

Dose: 1 drop tds of 0.5% solution (1% available for perioperative specialist use).

ARTHROTEC

Combination tablets of diclofenac with misoprostol (200 μg/tablet) to ↓GI SEs (esp PU/bleeds).

CI/Caution/SE/Interactions: see Diclofenac and Misoprostol.

Dose: 50 mg bd/tds po or 75 mg bd (prescribed as dose of diclofenac).

ASACOL see Mesalazine: 'new' aminosalicylate for UC with ↓SEs.

Available po (3–6 tablets of 400 mg per day in divided doses), as suppositories (0.75–1.5 g daily in divided doses) or as foam enemas (1–2 g daily).

ASPIRIN

NSAID. Inhibits COX-1 and COX-2. ⇒ ↓PG synthesis and anti-Pt action by inhibition of thromboxane A2.

Use: analgesic/anti-inflammatory/antipyrexial[1], IHD and thromboembolic CVA Px[2] and acute Rx[3].

CI: <16 years old (can ⇒ Reye's syndrome: liver/brain damage), **GI ulcers** (active or PHx of), bleeding disorders, gout, hypersensitivity (to any NSAID), **B**.

Caution: asthma, uncontrolled HTN, any allergic disease*, G6PD deficiency, dehydration, **L/R** (avoid if either severe)/**P/E**.

SE: bleeding (esp GI: ↑↑risk if also anticoagulated)**. Rarely ARF, blood disorders, hypersensitivity* (anaphylaxis, bronchospasm, skin reactions), ototoxic in OD.

Interactions: can ↑fx of sulphonylureas and methotrexate. **W+** (↑s anticoagulant fx and has additive fx on bleeding risk)**.

Dose: 300–900 mg 4–6-hourly (max 4 g/day)[1], 75 mg od[2], 300 mg stat[3].

Stop 7 days before surgery if significant bleeding is expected. If cardiac surgery or patient has ACS, consider continuing.

ATENOLOL

β-blocker: (mildly) cardioselective* ($\beta_1 > \beta_2$), ↑H_2O solubility
∴ ↓central fx** and ↑renal excretion***.
Use: HTN[1], angina[2], MI (w/in 12 h as early intervention)[3],
arrhythmias[4].
CI/Caution/SE/Interactions: see Propranolol, but ⇒
↓bronchospasm* (still avoid in asthma/COPD unless no other
choice) and ↓sleep disturbance/ nightmares**.
Dose: 25–50 mg od po[1]; 100 mg od po[2]; 5 mg iv over 5 min then
50 mg po 15 min later then start 50 mg bd 12 h later[3]; 50–100 mg od
po[4] (for iv doses see SPC/BNF). *Consider ↓ing dose in RF***.*

ATORVASTATIN/LIPITOR

HMG-CoA reductase inhibitor.
Use/CI/Caution/SE/Interactions: see Simvastatin.
Dose: initially 10 mg nocte (↑if necessary, at intervals ≥4 wks, to
max 80 mg).

iv ATROPINE (SULPHATE)

Muscarinic antagonist: blocks vagal SAN and AVN stimulation,
bronchodilates and ↓s oropharyngeal secretions.
Use: severe ↓HR (see algorithm in inside front cover) or HB[1], CPR[2]
(see ALS universal algorithm in inside back cover), organophosphate/
anticholinesterase* OD/poisoning[3] and specialist anaesthetic uses.
CI: (*do not apply if life threatening condition/CPR!*): glaucoma
(angle closure), MG (*unless anticholinesterase overdosage*, when
atropine is indicated*), paralytic ileus, pyloric stenosis, bladder neck
obstruction (e.g. ↑prostate).
Caution: Down's syndrome, gastro-oesophageal reflux, diarrhoea,
UC, acute MI, HTN, ↑HR (esp 2° to ↑T_4, cardiac insufficiency or
surgery), pyrexia, P/B/E.
SE: transient ↓HR (followed by ↑HR, palpitations, arrhythmias),
antimuscarinic fx (see p. 191), N&V, confusion (esp in elderly),
dizziness.
Dose: 0.3–1.0 mg iv[1]; 3 mg iv[2] (*if no iv/intraosseous access, give
6 mg with 10 ml saline via endotracheal tube*); 1–2 mg im/iv every

10–30 min[3] (every 5 min in severe cases) up to max 100 mg in 1st 24 h, until symptomatic response: skin flushes and dries, pupils dilate, HR ↑s).

ATROVENT see Ipratropium; bronchodilator for COPD/asthma

AUGMENTIN see Co-amoxiclav (amoxicillin + clavulanic acid) 375 or 625 mg tds po (1.2 g tds iv).

AZATHIOPRINE

Antiproliferative immunosuppressant: inhibits purine-salvage p'ways.
Use: prevention of transplant rejection, autoimmune disease (esp as steroid-sparing agent, but also maintenance Rx for SLE/vasculitis).
CI: hypersensitivity (to azathioprine *or mercaptopurine*), **B**.
Caution: L/R/P/E.
SE: **myelosuppression** (dose-dependent, ⇒ ↑infections, esp HZV), **hepatotoxicity**, **hypersensitivity reactions** (inc interstitial nephritis: *stop drug!*), **N&V&D** (esp initially), pancreatitis. Rarely cholestasis, alopecia, pneumonitis, risk of neoplasia.
Warn: immediately report infections or unexpected bruising/bleeding.
Monitor: FBC (initially ⩾weekly ↓ing to ⩾3-monthly), LFTs.
Interactions: fx ↑ by **allopurinol**, ACE-i, ARBs, trimethoprim (and septrin). fx↓ by rifampicin. **W−**.
Dose: 1–5 mg/kg daily[SPC/BNF] (preferably po as iv is very irritant).

> ☠Before starting Rx, screen for common gene defect of the enzyme TPMT (which metabolises azathioprine): if homozygote for defect avoid azathioprine; if heterozygote, ↓dose (esp if taking aminosalicylate derivatives, e.g. olsalazine, mesalazine or sulfasalazine). ☠

AZOPT see Brinzolamide; eye drops for glaucoma

AZT see Zidovudine; antiretroviral for HIV

BACLOFEN

Skeletal muscle relaxant: ↓s spinal reflexes, general CNS inhibition at ↑doses.

Use: spasticity, if chronic/severe, (esp 2° to MS or cord pathology).

CI: PU.

Caution: Ψ disorders, epilepsy, Hx of PU, Parkinson's, porphyria, DM, hypertonic bladder sphincter, respiratory/cerebrovascular disease, L/R/P/E.

SE: sedation, ↓muscle tone, nausea, urinary dysfunction, GI upset, ↓BP. Others rare: ↑spasticity (*stop drug!*), multiple neurological/Ψ symptoms, cardiac/hepatic/respiratory dysfunction.

Warn: may ↓skilled tasks (esp driving), ↑s fx of alcohol.

Interactions: fx ↑by TCAs. May ↑fx of antihypertensives.

Dose: 5 mg tds po (after food), ↑ to max of 100 mg/day. In severe cases, can give by intrathecal pump (see SPC/BNF).

Stop gradually over ⩾1–2 weeks to avoid withdrawal symptoms: hyperactivity, ↑spasticity, Ψ reactions, fits, autonomic dysfunction.

BACTROBAN see Mupirocin; topical antibiotic (esp for nasal MRSA). See local policy for infection control.

BALSALAZIDE

'New' aminosalicylate: prodrug of 5-ASA (↓sulphonamide SEs cf sulfasalazine).

Use/CI/Caution/SE/Warn/Monitor/Interactions: as mesalazine but **P/B** (CI instead of caution).

Dose: 2.25 g tds po in acute attack (for max 12 weeks). ↓to maintenance 1.5 g bd adjusted to response (max 6 g/day).

BECLOFORTE see Beclometasone (high dose at 250 μg/puff).

BECLOMETASONE

Inh corticosteroid: ↓s airway oedema and mucous secretions.

Use: chronic asthma not controlled by short-acting β_2 agonists alone (start at step 2 of BTS guidelines; see p. 152).

Caution: TB (inc quiescent).

SE: oral candidiasis (2° to immunosuppression: ↓d by rinsing mouth with H_2O after use), **hoarse voice**. Rarely glaucoma, hypersensitivity. ↑Doses may ⇒ adrenal suppression, Cushing's, ↓bone density, ↓growth (controversial).

Dose: 200–2000 µg daily inh (normally start at 200 µg bd). Use high-dose inhaler if daily requirements are >800 µg[SPC/BNF].

Rarely ⇒ paradoxical bronchospasm: can be prevented by switching from aerosol to dry powder forms or by using inh $β_2$ agonists.

BECOTIDE see Beclometasone (50, 100 or 200 µg/puff).

BENDROFLUMETHIAZIDE

Thiazide diuretic: ↓s Na^+ (and Cl^-) reabsorbtion from DCT ⇒ Na^+ and H_2O loss and stimulates K^+ excretion.

Use: oedema[1] (2° to HF or low–protein states), HTN[2] (in short term by ↓ing fluid volume and CO; in long term by ↓ing TPR), Px against renal stones in hypercalciuria[3].

CI: ↓K^+ (refractory to Rx), ↓Na^+, ↑Ca^{2+}, Addison's disease, ↑urate (if symptoms), **L/R** (if either severe, otherwise caution).

Caution: porphyria, and can worsen gout, DM or SLE, P/B/E.

SE: dehydration (esp in elderly), ↓**BP** (esp postural), ↓K^+, GI upset, **impotence**, ↓Na^+, alkalosis (with ↓Cl^-), ↓Mg^{++}, ↑Ca^{2+}, ↑urate/gout, ↑glucose, Δlipid metabolism (esp ↑cholesterol), rash, photosensitivity, blood disorders (inc ↓Pt, ↓NØ), pancreatitis, intrahepatic cholestasis, hyper-sensitivity reactions (inc severe respiratory and skin reactions).

Interactions: ↑s lithium levels. fx ↓by **NSAIDs** and oestrogens. If ↓ K^+ can ↑toxic fx of many drugs (esp digoxin, NSAIDs, corticosteroids and many antiarrhythmics). ↑risk of ↓Na^+ with carbamazepine and amphotericin.

Dose: initially 5–10 mg mane po[1], then ↓dose *frequency* (i.e. omit days) if possible; 2.5 mg od po[2,3] (little benefit from ↑doses).

BENZYLPENICILLIN (= PENICILLIN G)

Penicillin with poor po absorption ∴ only given im/iv: used mostly against streptococcal (esp *S. pneumoniae*) and neisserial (esp *N. gonorrhoeae*, *N. meningitidis*) infections.

Use: severe skin infections (esp cellulitis, wound infections, gas gangrene) in conjunction with other agents (see p. 148), meningitis, endocarditis, ENT infections.

CI: penicillin hypersensitivity (NB: cross-reactivity with cefalosporins possible).

Caution: Hx of allergy, **R***.

SE: hypersensitivity (inc fever, arthralgia, rashes, urticaria, angioedema, anaphylaxis, serum sickness-like reactions, haemolytic ↓Hb, interstitial nephritis), **diarrhoea** (rarely AAC). Rarely blood disorders (↓Pt, ↓NØ, coagulation disorders), CNS toxicity (inc convulsions, esp at ↑doses or if RF*). ↑doses can ⇒ ↓K⁺ (and ↓Na⁺).

Interactions: levels ↑d by probenecid. ↑risk of rash with allopurinol. Can ↓fx of OCP.

Dose: 1.2 g qds iv (or im/ivi). If very severe, give 2.4 g every 4 h (only as iv/ivi).

BETAGAN see Levobunolol; β-blocker eye drops for glaucoma.

BETAHISTINE/SERC

Histamine analogue (H_1 antagonism and H_3 antagonism): ↑s middle-ear microcirculation ⇒ ↓endolymphatic pressure.

Use: Ménière's disease (if tinnitus, vertigo or hearing loss).

CI: phaeo.

Caution: asthma, Hx of PU, P/B.

SE: GI upset. Rarely headache, rash, pruritus.

Dose: 16 mg tds po (maintenance normally 24–48 mg/day).

BETAMETHASONE CREAM (0.1%)

'Potent' strength topical corticosteroid (rarely used as weaker 0.05% or 0.025% preparations).

BETNOVATE see Betamethasone cream 0.1% (potent strength).
Available as Betnovate RD (moderate strength) 0.025%.

BEZAFIBRATE
Fibrate (lipid-lowering): $\Rightarrow$ ↓**TG**, ↓LDL, ↑HDL by stimulating
lipoprotein lipase ($\Rightarrow$ ↓conversion of VLDL/TG to LDL and
$\Rightarrow$ ↑LDL clearance from circulation). Also $\Rightarrow$ (mild) ↓cholesterol.
Use: hyperlipidaemias (esp if ↑TG ∴ types IIa/b, III, IV, V).
CI: gallbladder disease, PBC, ↓albumin (esp nephrotic syndrome),
R*/L (if either severe; otherwise caution), **P/B**.
Caution: ↓T_4 (needs to be corrected).
SE: GI upset, ↓**appetite**, ↑**gallstones**, **myositis** (rarer but
important: ↑risk if RF*). Also impotence, rash (inc pruritus,
urticaria), headache. Rarer: dizziness, vertigo, fatigue, hair loss,
blood disorders (↓Hb, ↓WCC, ↓Pt).
Interactions: 💀'statins'. ↑risk of myositis. 💀 ↑s fx of
antidiabetics. ↑risk of hepatotoxicity with MAOIs. Can ↑renal
toxicity of ciclosporin. **W+.**
Dose: 200 mg tds po (after food). MR 400 mg od preps available[BNF].

BICARBONATE see Sodium bicarbonate

▼BISOPROLOL
β-blocker, cardioselective ($\beta_1 > \beta_2$).
Use: HTN[1], angina[2], HF[3].
CI/Caution/SE/Interactions: as propranolol, but also CI in HF
needing inotropes or if SAN block; caution if psoriasis.
Dose: 10 mg od po[1,2] (maintenance 5–20 mg od); initially 1.25 mg
od po[3] (↑ing slowly to max 10 mg od)[SPC/BNF].
Consider ↓ing doses in RF and LF.

BOWEL PREPARATIONS
Bowel-cleansing solutions for preparation for GI surgery/Ix.
CI: GI obstruction/ulceration/perforation, ileus, gastric retention,
toxic megacolon/colitis, **H**.

Caution: UC, DM, heart disease, reflux oesophagitis, ↑risk of regurgitation/aspiration (e.g. ↓swallow/gag reflex/GCS), R/P.
SE: nausea, bloating, abdominal pains, vomiting.
Dose: see Citramag, Fleet (Phospho-soda), Klean-prep, Picolax.

BRICANYL see Terbutaline (inh β₂ agonist for asthma). Various delivery devices available$^{SPC/BNF}$.

BRIMONIDINE EYE DROPS/ALPHAGAN
Topical α₂ agonist: ↓s aqueous humour production ∴ ↓s IOP.
Use: open-angle glaucoma, ocular HTN (2nd-line if β-blocker drops are unsuitable or control IOP inadequately).
Caution: postural ↓BP, Raynaud's, cardiovascular disease (esp IHD), cerebral insufficiency, depression*, P/B/R/L.
SE: sedation, headache, blurred vision, dry mouth/nose, **local reactions** (esp discomfort, pruritus, hyperaemia, follicular conjunctivitis). Rarely HTN, palpitations, depression*, hypersensitivity.
Interactions: ☠MAOIs, TCAs, mianserin (or other antidepressants affecting NA transmission) are CI.☠
Dose: 1 drop bd of 0.2% solution.

BRINZOLAMIDE/AZOPT
Topical carbonic anhydrase inhibitor for glaucoma. Similar to dorzolamide (↓s aqueous humour production).
Dose: 1 drop bd/tds (of 10 mg/ml solution).

BROMOCRIPTINE
DA agonist; ↓s pituitary release of prolactin/growth hormone.
Use: parkinsonism if L-dopa insufficient/not tolerated, NMS, endocrine disorders (if prolactin or growth hormone related).
CI: toxaemia of pregnancy, hypersensitivity to ergot alkaloids, uncontrolled HTN. Also HTN/IHD postpartum or in puerperium.
Caution: cardiovascular disease, porphyria, Raynaud's disease, serious Ψ disorders (esp psychosis), P/B.

SE: GI upset, postural $\downarrow$**BP** (esp initially and if $\uparrow$alcohol intake), **behavioural Δs** (confusional states, Ψ disorders), $\uparrow$**sleep** (sudden onset/daytime). Rarely but seriously **fibrosis***: pulmonary**, cardiac, retroperitoneal*** (can $\Rightarrow$ ARF).
Warn: of $\uparrow$sleep. Report persistent cough** or chest/abdo pain.
Monitor: ESR*, U&Es***, CXR**.
Interactions: levels $\uparrow$by ery-/clari-thromycin and octreotide.
Dose: 1–30 mg/day[SPC/BNF].

BUCCASTEM Prochlorperazine (antiemetic) buccal tablets: absorbed rapidly from under top lip $\therefore$ do not need to be swallowed and retained in stomach for absorption if N&V.
Dose: 3–6 mg bd.

BUDESONIDE

Inh corticosteroid similar to beclometasone but stronger (approximately double the strength per microgram).
Dose: 200–800 μg bd inh (aerosol or powder) or 1–2 mg bd neb.

BUMETANIDE

Loop diuretic: inhibits Na^+/K^+ pump in ascending loop of Henle.
Use/CI/Caution/SE/Monitor/Interactions: as furosemide; also can $\Rightarrow$ myalgia at $\uparrow$doses.
Dose: 1 mg mane po (500 μg may suffice in elderly), $\uparrow$ing if required (5 mg/24 h usually sufficient; $\uparrow$by adding a lunchtime dose, then $\uparrow$ing each dose). 1–2 mg im/iv (repeat after 20 min if required). 2–5 mg ivi over 30–60 min.

NB: give iv in severe oedema; bowel oedema $\Rightarrow$ $\downarrow$po absorption.

▼BUPROPION (= AMFEBUTAMONE)/ZYBAN

NA and to lesser extent DA reuptake inhibitor (NDRI) developed as antidepressant, but also $\uparrow$s success of giving up smoking.
Use: (adjunct to) smoking cessation[NICE].
CI: CNS tumour, acute alcohol/benzodiazepine withdrawal, Hx of seizures*, eating disorders, bipolar disorder, **L** (if severe cirrhosis)/**P/B**.

Caution: if ↑risk of seizures*: alcohol abuse, Hx of head trauma and DM, R/E.

SE: seizures*, insomnia (and other CNS reactions, e.g. anxiety, agitation, depression, headaches, tremor, dizziness). Also ↑HR, AV block, ↑ or ↓BP**, hypersensitivity (inc severe skin reactions), GI upset, ↑Wt, mild antimuscarinic fx (esp **dry mouth**; see p. 191 for others).

Monitor: BP**.

Interactions: ↓P450 ∴ many interactions, but importantly **CNS drugs, esp if ↓seizure threshold***, e.g. antidepressants (☠MAOIs are CI☠), antimalarials, antipsychotics (esp risperidone), quinolones, sedating antihistamines, systemic corticosteroids, theophyllines, tramadol. Ritonavir ⇒ ↑toxic fx.

Dose: 150 mg od for 6 days then 150 mg bd for max 9 wks (↓dose if elderly or ↑seizure risk [SPC/BNF]). Start 1–2 wks before target date of stopping smoking.

BURINEX Bumetanide 1-mg tablets. Also available as K⁺-conserving preparations: Burinex A (1 mg bumetanide + 5 mg amiloride) and Burinex K (0.5 mg bumetanide + 7.7 mmol K⁺).

BUSCOPAN see Hyoscine butylbromide; GI antispasmodic.

CACIT see Calcium carbonate

CACIT D3 Calcium carbonate + low dose vitamin D₃.
Use: Px of vitamin D deficiency.
Dose: 1 tablet od (= 12.6 mmol Ca²⁺ + 11 μg cholecalciferol).

CALCICHEW see Calcium carbonate

CALCICHEW D3 Calcium carbonate + low dose vitamin D₃.
Use: Px of vitamin D deficiency.

Dose: 1 tablet od. Each tablet = 12.6 mmol Ca^{2+} + 5 µg vit D_3 (cholecalciferol) or 10 µg vit D_3 in 'forte' preparations.

CALCITONIN

Synthetic hormone (normally produced by C cells of thyroid): binds to specific osteoclast receptors $\Rightarrow$ ↓resorption of bone and ↓Ca^{2+}. Its fx are specific to abnormal (high-turnover) bone.

Use: ↑Ca^{2+} (esp dt malignancy; also ↓s bone metastases pain), Paget's disease (↓s pain and neurological symptoms, e.g. deafness), rarely for Px/Rx of postmenopausal osteoporosis.

CI: ↓Ca^{2+}.

Caution: Hx of *any* allergy, R/H/P/B.

SE: GI upset (esp N&V), **flushing**, ↑**urinary frequency**, taste and sensory Δ, hypersensitivity (inc anaphylaxis), local inflammation.

Dose: see BNF/SPC.

CALCIUM CARBONATE

Use: osteoporosis, ↓Ca^{2+}, ↑PO_4 (esp 2° to RF; binds PO_4 in gut $\Rightarrow$ ↓absorption).

CI: conditions assoc with ↑Ca^{2+} (in serum or urine).

Caution: sarcoid, Hx of kidney stones, phenylketonuria, R.

SE: GI upset, ↑Ca^{2+} (serum or urine), ↓HR, arrhythmias.

Interactions: fx ↑by thiazides, fx ↓by corticosteroids, ↓s absorption of tetracyclines (give ≥2 h before or 6 h after) and bisphosphonates.

Dose: as required up to 40 mmol/day in osteoporosis if ↓dietary intake, e.g. Calcichew (standard 12.6-mmol or 'forte' 25-mmol tablets), Cacit (12.6-mmol tablets), Calcium 500 (12.5-mmol tablets) or Adcal (15-mmol tablets).

CALCIUM CHLORIDE

Ca^{2+} for emergency iv use: mostly CPR as $\Rightarrow$ ↑venous irritation cf calcium gluconate. Can also use for severe ↓Ca^{2+} or ↑K^+.

CI: VF, conditions assoc with ↑Ca^{2+} (in serum or urine).

SE: GI upset, $\uparrow Ca^{2+}$, $\downarrow$HR, $\downarrow$BP, arrhythmias.

Dose: available as syringes of 10 ml of 10% solution (= total of 6.8 mmol Ca^{2+}). Give iv no quicker than 1 ml/min (otherwise can $\Rightarrow$ arrhythmias) as per indication and clinical/e'lyte response.

e.g. Min-i-Jet: often in crash trolleys if iv Ca^{2+} needed urgently.

CALCIUM + ERGOCALCIFEROL tablets of 2.4 mmol Ca^{2+} + low-dose (10 µg) ergocalciferol (= calciferol = vitamin D_2).

Use: Px of vitamin D deficiency.

CI/Caution/SE: see Ergocalciferol.

Dose: 1 tablet od.

CALCIUM GLUCONATE

iv preparation of Ca^{2+} (also available po, but used rarely).

Use: $\downarrow Ca^{2+}$ (if severe)[1], $\uparrow K^+$ ($\downarrow$s arrhythmias: 'cardioprotective', see p. 208)[2], $\uparrow Mg^{2+}$.

CI/SE: as calcium chloride.

Dose: 10 ml of 10% iv over 2 min (= total of 2.2 mmol Ca^{2+})[1,2], repeating if necessary according to clinical and electrolyte response; consider following with ivi[1].

CALCIUM RESONIUM

Polystyrene sulphonate ion-exchange resin.

Use: mild/moderate $\uparrow K^+$ (not for *initial** Mx of severe $\uparrow K^+$).

CI: obstructive bowel disease, diseases likely to $\uparrow Ca^{2+}$ ($\uparrow$PTH, multiple myeloma, sarcoid, metastatic cancer), $K^+ < 5$ mmol/l.

Caution: P/B.

SE: GI upset (esp constipation; often need Px of 10–20 ml lactulose), $\downarrow K^+$, $\downarrow Mg^{2+}$, $\uparrow Ca^{2+}$ and Na^+ retention.

Dose: 15 g tds/qds po. NB: takes 24–48 h to work*. Also available as 30-g enemas (rarely $\Rightarrow$ rectal ulceration and colonic necrosis: needs cleansing enema first and washout afterwards; see SPC).

CALPOL Paracetamol (paediatric) suspension.

Dose: according to age; all doses can be given up to max frequency qds (min dose spacing = 4 h): 3 months–1 year 60–120 mg, 1–5 years 120–250 mg, 6–12 years 250–500 mg, >12 years 500–1000 mg (= adult dose).

Two strengths available: 'standard' (120 mg/5 ml) and '6 plus' (250 mg/5 ml).

CANDESARTAN/AMIAS
Angiotensin II antagonist.
Use: HTN[1], HF[2].
CI: cholestasis, **L** (if severe)/**P/B**.
Caution/SE/Interactions: see Losartan.
Dose: initially 8 mg od[1] (2 mg if LF, 4 mg if RF/intravascular volume depletion) ↑ing at 4 wk intervals if necessary to max of 32 mg od; initially 4 mg od[2] ↑ing at intervals ≥2wks to 'target dose' of 32 mg od (or max tolerated).

CANESTEN Clotrimazole 1% cream: antifungal, esp for vaginal candida infections (thrush). Also available as powder, solution and spray for hairy areas.
Dose: apply bd/tds.

CAPTOPRIL
ACE-i: short-acting; largely replaced by longer-acting (od) drugs.
Use: HTN, HF, post-MI, and diabetic nephropathy (i.e. consistent proteinuria).
CI: renovascular disease* (known or suspected bilateral RAS), angioedema/other hypersensitivity 2° to ACEi, porphyria, **P**.
Caution: symptomatic aortic stenosis, Hx of idiopathic or hereditary angioedema, **L/R/B/E**.
SE: ↓**BP** (esp with 1st dose, if HF, dehydrated or on diuretics, dialysis or ↓Na$^+$ diet ∴ *take at night*), **RF***, **dry cough**, ↑**K**$^+$, **hypersensitivity** (esp rashes and **angioedema**), Δ taste, upper respiratory tract symptoms (inc sore throat/sinusitis/rhinitis),

GI upset, Δ LFTs (rarely cholestatic jaundice/hepatitis), pancreatitis, blood disorders, many non-specific neuro symptoms.
Monitor: U&Es, esp baseline and *2 wks after starting**.
Interactions: fx ↓d by NSAIDs (also ⇒ ↑risk RF*). **Diuretics**, TCAs and antipsychotics ⇒ risk of ↓↓BP. ↑s fx of **lithium** (and antidiabetics).
Dose: 6.25–75 mg bd po$^{SPC/BNF}$.

☠Beware if on other drugs that ↑K⁺, e.g. amiloride, spirono-lactone, triamterene, ARBs and ciclosporin. Don't give with oral K⁺ supplements – inc dietary salt substitutes. ☠

CARBAMAZEPINE/TEGRETOL
Antiepileptic, mood stabiliser, analgesic; ↓s synaptic transmission.
Use: epilepsy[1], Px bipolar disorder[2] (if unresponsive to lithium), neuralgia[3] (esp post-herpetic, trigeminal and DM-related).
CI: unpaced AV conduction dfx, Hx of BM suppression, porphyria.
Caution: cardiac disease, Hx skin disorders or haematological drug reactions, glaucoma, **L/R**, **P** (⇒ neural tube dfx* ∴ ⇒ folate Px and screen for dfx), **B**.
Dose-related SEs: dizziness, vertigo, ataxia, visual Δ (esp double vision): control by ↓ing dose, Δ dose times/ spacing or use of MR preparations**. **Other SEs: skin reactions, blood disorders** (esp ↓WCC*** – often transient, esp initially), **GI upset, ↓Na⁺** (inc SIADH), **drowsiness**, HF, arrhythmias, AV block, pulmonary hypersensitivity. Many rarer SEs$^{SPC/BNF}$.
Monitor: serum levels (optimum therapeutic range = 4–12 mg/l), U&Es, LFTs, FBC***.
Warn: driving may be impaired, and watch for signs of liver/skin/ haematological disease.
Interactions: ↑P450 ∴ many (see SPC/BNF); most importantly, fx are ↑d by **ery-/clari-thromycin**, isoniazid, verapamil and diltiazem; and it ↓s fx of **OCP** (NB: *carbamazepine is teratogenic!**), **corticosteroids**, other antiepileptics (NB: *can also autoinduce!*).
☠CI with MAOIs.☠ **W–**.

Dose: initially 100–200 mg od/bd ($\uparrow$slowly to max of 1.6 g/day[2,3] or 2 g/day[1]). (MR forms** available[SPC/BNF])

CARBIMAZOLE

Thionamide antithyroid: peroxidase inhibitor; stops $I^- \Rightarrow I_2$ and $\therefore \downarrow$s T_3/T_4 production. ?Also immunosuppressive fx.
Use: $\uparrow T_4$.
Caution: L, P/B (can cause fetal/neonatal goitre/$\downarrow T_4$ $\therefore$ use min dose to control symptoms and monitor neonatal development closely – 'block-and-replace' regimen $\therefore$ not suitable).
SE: hypersensitivity: rash and **pruritus** (if symptoms not tolerated or not eased by antihistamines, switch to propylthiouracil), fever, arthralgia. Also GI disturbance (esp nausea), headache, rash and pruritis. Rarely hepatic dysfunction, alopecia, blood disorders – esp **agranulocytosis*** (0.5%) and $\downarrow$WCC (often transient and benign).
Warn/monitor: see box below.
Dose: 15–60 mg/day in 2–3 divided doses ($\downarrow$dose once euthyroid; maintenance dose usually 5–15 mg od, unless on 'block-and-replace' regimen, where $\uparrow$d doses are maintained). *Normally give for only 12–18 months. Remission often occurs; if not, other Rx (e.g. surgery/radioiodine) may be needed.*

> ☠**Agranulocytosis:** warn patient to report immediately signs/symptoms of infection (esp sore throat, but also fever, malaise, mouth ulcers, bruising and non-specific illness). If suspect infection, do FBC (routine screening unhelpful as can occur rapidly). Stop drug if clinical or laboratory evidence of $\downarrow$NØ*.☠

CARVEDILOL

β-blocker: non-selective but also blocks α_1 $\therefore \Rightarrow$ arterial vasodilation.
Use: HF[1] (if stable). Less commonly for angina[2] and HTN[3].
CI/Caution: as propranolol, plus **L**. Also **H** if severe *and chronic* HF (caution in severe *and non-chronic* HF, and avoid if acute or decompensated HF needing iv inotropes).
SE: as propranolol, but worse postural $\downarrow$BP.
Interactions: as propranolol, but can $\uparrow$levels of ciclosporin.

Dose: initially 3.125 mg bd[1] (↑at intervals ⩾2 wks to max of 25–50 mg bd); initially 12.5 mg bd[2]/od[3] (can ↑ to 50 mg/day). Before ↑ing dose, check HF and renal function not worsening.

CEFACLOR

Oral 2nd-generation cephalosporin.

Use: mild respiratory infections, UTIs, external infections (skin/soft-tissue infections, sinusitis, otitis media), esp in pregnancy* (is one of the safest antibiotics) or dt *H. influenzae*.

CI: cephalosporin hypersensitivity.

Caution: penicillin hypersensitivity (10% also allergic to cephalosporins), **R** (↓doses may be required; threshold depends on individual cephalosporin[SPC/BNF]), **P/B** (but appropriate to use*).

SE: GI upset (esp N&D, rarely AAC), **allergy** (anaphylaxis, fever, arthralgia, skin reactions (inc severe)), **ARF**, **interstitial nephritis** (reversible), hepatic dysfunction, blood disorders, CNS disturbance (inc headache).

Interactions: levels ↑by probenecid, mild **W⁺**.

Dose: 250 mg tds po (500 mg tds in severe infections; max 4 g/day). Cephalosporins can ⇒ false-positive Coombs' and urinary glucose tests.

CEFALEXIN

Oral 1st-generation cephalosporin.

Use/CI/Caution/SE/Interactions: see Cefaclor.

Dose: 250 mg qds or 500 mg bd/tds po (↑ in severe infections to max 1.5 g qds). For Px of UTI, give 125 mg po nocte.

CEFOTAXIME

Parenteral 3rd-generation cephalosporin.

Use: severe infections, esp meningitis and sepsis 2° to hospital-acquired pneumonia, UTI, pyelonephritis, soft-tissue infections.

CI/Caution/SE/Interactions: see Cefaclor, but can also rarely ⇒ arrhythmias if given as rapid iv injection.

Dose: 1 g bd im/iv/ivi (↑ing to max of 3 g qds if needed).

CEFRADINE

Oral or parenteral 1st-generation cephalosporin.

Use: as cefaclor, plus preoperative Px[1].

CI/Caution/SE/Interactions: see Cefaclor.

Dose: po: 250–500 mg qds *or* 0.5–1 g bd (max 1 g qds). **im/iv/ivi:** 0.5–1 g qds (max 2 g qds). 1–2 g im/iv at induction[1].

CEFTAZIDIME

Parenteral 3rd-generation cephalosporin: good against *Pseudomonas*.

Use: see Cefotaxime (often reserved for ITU setting).

CI/Caution/SE/Interactions: see Cefaclor.

Dose: 1 g tds im/iv/ivi, ↑ing (with care in elderly) to 2 g tds iv (not im, where max single dose is 1 g) if life-threatening, e.g. meningitis, immunocompromised.

CEFTRIAXONE

Parenteral 3rd-generation cephalosporin.

Use: as cefotaxime, plus preoperative Px[1].

CI/Caution/SE/Interactions: as Cefaclor, plus **L** (if coexistent RF), **R** (if severe), caution if dehydrated, young or immobile (can precipitate in urine or gallbladder). Rarely ⇒ pancreatitis and ↑PT.

Dose: 1 g od im/iv/ivi (max 4 g/day); 1–2 g im/iv/ivi at induction[1]. Max im dose = 1 g per site; if total >1 g, give at divided sites.

CEFUROXIME

Parenteral and oral 2nd-generation cephalosporin: good for some Gram-negative infections (*H. influenzae*, *N. gonorrhoeae*) and better than 3rd-generation cephalosporins for Gram-positive infections (esp *S. aureus*).

Use: *po:* respiratory infections[1], UTIs[2], pyelonephritis[3]; *iv:* severe infections[4], preoperative Px[5].

CI/Caution/SE/Interactions: see Cefaclor.

Dose: 250–500 mg bd po[1]; 125 mg bd po[2]; 250 mg bd po[3]; 750 mg tds/qds iv/im[4] (1.5 g tds/qds iv in very severe infections and

3 g tds if meningitis); 1.5 g iv at induction (+750 mg iv/im tds for 24 h if high-risk procedure)[5].

CELECOXIB/CELEBREX
NSAID with selective inhibition of COX-2 ∴ ↓GI SEs (COX-1-mediated). *Provides no Px against IHD/CVA* (unlike aspirin).
Use: osteo/rheumatoid arthritis[NICE]. Beneficial GI fx (↓bleeding), lost if on aspirin ∴ don't use together.
CI: IHD, cerebrovascular disease, active bleeding/Pu, PVD hypersensitivity to any NSAID (inc asthma, angioedema, urticaria, acute rhinitis, nasal polyps), *sulphonamide* hypersensitivity, IBD, **L/R** (if either severe; otherwise caution) **H/P/B**.
Caution: Hx of PU/GI bleeding, ↑cardiovascular risk (e.g. HTN, DM, ↑lipids, PVD, smokers), oedema (of any cause), **E**.
SE/Interactions: as ibuprofen, but ↓GI ulceration/bleeding. Also can → peripheral oedema (even if no predisposing cause), MI, HF, GI upset, HTN, back pain, headache, dizziness and rarely CVA. Also ↑risk of RF with ACE-i, ARB or ciclosporin and can ↑levels of TCAs, SSRIs, neuroleptics and antiarrhythmics.
Dose: 100–200 mg bd po.

> **COX-2 inhibitors and ↑risk of cardiovascular complications:** CSM advises assessment of cardiovascular risk and use in preference to other NSAIDs only if at ↑↑risk of GI ulcer, perforation or bleeding. Patients on COX-2 inhibitor with IHD or cerebrovascular disease should be switched to alternative ASAP.

CEPH– see CEF–

CETIRIZINE/ZIRTEK
Non-sedating antihistamine: selective peripheral H_1 antagonist.
Use: allergy: symptomatic relief from (esp hay fever, urticaria).
CI: P/B.
Caution: epilepsy, ↑prostate/urinary retention, glaucoma, pyloroduodenal obstruction, **R** (halve doses)/**L**.
SE: mild antimuscarinic fx (see p. 191), very mild sedation, headache.

Warn: may impair driving.
Dose: 10 mg od (or 5 mg bd) po.

CHARCOAL

Binds and ↓s absorption of tablets/poisons.
Use: ODs (up to 1 h post-ingestion; longer if MR/SR preparations or antimuscarinic drugs. See pp. 210–11).
Caution: corrosive poisons, ↓GI motility (can ⇒ obstruction), ↓GCS (risk of aspiration, unless endotracheal tube in situ).
Dose: 50 g. Give once for paracetamol, salicylates and TCAs. Repeated doses (every 4 h) often needed for barbiturates, carbamazepine, phenytoin, digoxin, dapsone, paraquat, quinine, theophylline and MR/SR preparations.

CHLORAMPHENICOL iv (and po)

Broad-spectrum antibiotic: inhibits bacterial protein synthesis (∴ 'static'); very potent action, but SEs limit use.
Use: severe infections (esp *H. influenzae*) and rickettsiae (e.g. typhoid).
CI: porphyria **P/B**.
Caution: **L/E** (↓dose/check levels*), **R**.
SE: blood disorders (inc aplastic ↓Hb), neuritis (peripheral, optic), GI upset, hepatotoxicity, hypersensitivity, stomatitis, glossitis.
Monitor: FBC, serum drug levels* pre-dose (trough) and 1 h post-dose (peak).
Interactions: ↑s fx of sulphonylureas, phenytoin, ciclosporin and tacrolimus. ↑risk of agranulocytosis with clozapine. Phenobarbital and primidone ↓s its fx. **W+**.
Dose: 50 mg/kg/day in 4 divided doses iv (or rarely po), ↑ing to 100 mg/kg/day if life-threatening infection.

CHLORAMPHENICOL EYE DROPS

Topical preparation, with no significant systemic fx, for superficial bacterial eye infections. Can rarely ⇒ aplastic anaemia.
Dose: 1 × 0.5% drop to affected eye(s) at least 2-hourly (↓once infection controlled, continue after healed for 48 h). Can give as

1% ointment applied tds/qds (or nocte only if taking drops in daytime as well).

CHLORDIAZEPOXIDE
Benzodiazepine, long-acting.
Use: anxiety (esp in alcohol withdrawal).
CI/Caution/SE/Interactions: see Diazepam.
Dose: 10 mg tds po, ↑ing if required to max of 100 mg/day. ↓dose in elderly, ↑dose if benzodiazepine-resistant or in initial Rx of alcohol withdrawal (see p. 161 for reducing regimen).

CHLORHEXIDINE
Disinfectant mouthwash or solution for skin cleansing before invasive procedures and bladder washout.

CHLOROQUINE
Antimalarial: inhibits protein synthesis and DNA/RNA polymerases.
Use: malaria Px[1] (only as Rx[2] if 'benign' spp (i.e. *P.ovale/vivax/malariae*); *P.falciparum* often resistant). Rarely for RA, SLE.
Caution: G6PD deficiency, severe GI disorders, can worsen psoriasis and MG, neurological disorders (esp epilepsy*), **L** (avoid other hepatotoxic drugs), **R/P**.
SE: GI upset, headache (mild, transient), **visual Δ** (rarely retinopathy**), **seizures***, hypersensitivity/skin reactions (inc pigment Δs), hair loss. Rarely **BM suppression**, cardiomyopathy. Arrhythmias common in OD.
Monitor: FBC, vision** (+ ophthalmology review if on long-term Rx).
Interactions: absorption ↓by antacids. ↑risk of arrhythmias with amiodarone and moxifloxacin. ↑risk of convulsions with mefloquine. ↑s levels of digoxin and ciclosporin. ↓s levels of praziquantel.
Dose: *Px[1]*: 300 mg once weekly *as base (specify on prescription: do not confuse with salt doses)*. Used mostly in conjunction with other drugs, depending on local resistance patterns[SPC/BNF].
Rx[2]: see p. 146.

CHLORPHEN(IR)AMINE/PIRITON

Antihistamine: H_1 antagonist (peripheral *and central* ∴ sedating).
Use: allergies[1] (esp drug reactions, hay fever, urticaria),
anaphylaxis[2] (inc blood transfusion reaction[3]).
CI: hypersensitivity to any antihistamine.
Caution: pyloroduodenal obstruction, urinary retention/↑prostate,
thyrotoxicosis, asthma, bronch-itis/-iectasis, severe HTN/cardiovascular
disease, glaucoma, epilepsy, **R/L/P/B**.
SE: **drowsiness** (rarely paradoxical stimulation), **antimuscarinic** fx
(esp dry mouth; see p. 191), GI upset, arrhythmias, ↓BP, skin and
hypersensitivity reactions (inc bronchospasm, photosensitivity).
Warn: driving may be impaired.
Interactions: Can ↑phenytoin levels. ☠**MAOIs*** can ⇒ ↑↑
antimuscarinic fx (SPC says chlorphenamine CI if MAOI given
w/in 2 wks but evidence unclear).☠
Dose: 4 mg 4–6-hourly po[1]; 10 mg iv over 1 min[2] (can ↑ to 20 mg,
max 40 mg/24 h); 10–20 mg sc[3] (max 40 mg/24 h).

CHLORPROMAZINE

Phenothiazine ('typical') antipsychotic: dopamine antagonist
($D_{1\&3} > D_{2\&4}$). Also blocks serotonin ($5HT_{2A}$), histamine (H_1),
adrenergic ($\alpha_{1>2}$) and muscarinic receptors, causing many SEs.
Use: schizophrenia[1], acute sedation[2] (inc mania, severe anxiety,
violent behaviour), intractable hiccups[3].
CI: CNS depression (inc coma), Hx of blood dyscrasias, severe
cardiovascular disease.
Caution: Parkinson's, drugs that ↑QTc, epilepsy, MG, phaeo,
glaucoma (angle-closure), ↑prostate, severe respiratory disease,
jaundice, blood disorders, predisposition to postural ↓BP, ↑or
↓temperature. Avoid direct sunlight (⇒ photosensitivity), **L/R/H/P/B/E**.
Class SE: **sedation**, **extrapyramidal fx** (see pp. 192–3), **antimuscarinic
fx** (see p. 191), **seizures**, ↑Wt, ↓BP (esp postural), ECG Δs (↑QTc),
arrhythmias, endocrine fx (menstrual Δs, galactorrhoea, gynaecomastia,
sexual dysfunction), ΔLFTs/jaundice, blood disorders (inc agranulocytosis,
↓WCC), ↓ or ↑temperature (esp in elderly), rash/↑pigmentation,
neuroleptic malignant syndrome.

Warn: avoid alcohol and direct sunlight, ↓s skilled tasks (inc driving).
Monitor: FBC, BP.
Interactions: fx ↑d by TCAs (esp antimuscarinic fx), lithium (esp extrapyramidal fx +/− neurotoxicity), cimetidine and β-blockers (esp arrhythmias with sotalol; propranolol fx also ↑d by chlorpromazine).
Dose: 25–300 mg tds po$^{SPC/BNF}$ (↓dose in elderly: 10 mg od may suffice); 25–50 mg tds/qds im (painful, and may ⇒ ↓BP/↑HR).

CICLOSPORIN

Calcineurin inhibitor: ⇒ ↓IL-2-mediated LØ proliferation.
Use: immunosuppression (esp nephrotic syndrome and post-transplant).
CI (*only apply if given for nephrotic syndrome*)**:** uncontrolled infection or HTN, malignancy.
Caution: HTN, ↑urate, porphyria, drugs that ↑K$^+$, **L/R/P/B/E.**
SE: nephrotoxicity and **tremor** (both dose-related), ↑BP, hepatotoxicity, GI upset, biochemical Δs (↑K$^+$, ↑urate/gout, ↓Mg^{++}, ↑cholesterol). Rarely neuromuscular symptoms, HUS, neoplasms (esp lymphoma).
Warn: hypertrichosis, gingival hypertrophy, burning sensation in hands and feet.
Monitor: levels, LFTs, U&Es, Mg^{++}, lipids, BP.
Interactions: metabolised by **P450**, ∴ many, particularly antibacterials and antifungals$^{SPC/BNF}$ (cephalosporins and penicillins OK). Levels esp ↓by phenytoin, carbamazepine, phenobarbital, St John's wort, rifampicin, orlistat, ticlopidine and octreotide. Levels esp ↑by ery-/clari-thromycin, keto-/flu-/itra-conazole, protease inhibitors, diltiazem, nicardipine, verapamil, metoclopramide, amiodarone, allopurinol, dazazol, ursodeoxycholic acid, corticosteroids and OCP. Can ↑levels of digoxin and diclofenac. Nephrotoxic and myotoxic drugs can become more so.
Dose: specialist use$^{SPC/BNF}$. Must prescribe by brand name (Neoral, Sandimmun or SangCya) as have different bioavailabilities and changing brands can ∴ ↓immunosuppression or ↑toxicity.

☠ Check all new drugs for interactions before prescribing if on ciclosporin: ↑d levels ⇒ toxicity; ↓d levels may ⇒ rejection. ☠

CIMETIDINE

As ranitidine, but ↑↑interactions (↓**P450** & **W+**) and ↑gynaecomastia ∴ prescribed rarely. Dose: 400 mg bd (can ↑ to 4 hrly[SPC/BNF]).

CIPROFLOXACIN

(Fluoro)quinolone antibiotic: inhibits DNA gyrase; 'cidal' with broad spectrum, but particularly good for Gram-negative infections.
Use: GI infections[1] (esp salmonella, shigella, campylobacter), **respiratory infections** (non-pneumococcal pneumonias[2], esp *Pseudomonas*). Also GU infections (esp UTIs[3], acute uncomplicated cystitis in women[4], gonorrhoea), 1st-line initial Rx of anthrax.
CI: hypersensitivity to any quinolone, **P/B**.
Caution: seizures (inc Hx of, or predisposition to), MG (can worsen), G6PD deficiency, children/adolescents (theoretical risk of arthropathy), avoid ↑urine pH/dehydration*, **R**.
SE: GI upset (esp N&D, rarely AAC), **neuro-Ψ fx** (esp confusion, **seizures**; also headache, dizziness, hallucinations, sleep and mood Δs), **tendinitis ± rupture** (esp if elderly or taking steroids), **hypersensitivity** (rash, pruritis, fever). Rarely hepatotoxicity, RF/interstitial nephritis, crystaluria*, blood disorders, skin reactions (inc photosensitivity**, SJS, TEN).
Warn: avoid UV light**, avoid ingesting Fe- and Zn-containing products (e.g. antacids***). May impair skilled tasks/driving.
Interactions: ↑s levels of theophyllines; NSAIDs ⇒ ↑risk of seizures; ↑s nephrotoxicity of ciclosporin; FeSO$_4$ and antacids*** ⇒ ↓ciprofloxacin absorption (give 2 h before or 6 h after ciprofloxacin), **W+**.
Dose: 250–750 mg bd po, 100–400 mg bd ivi (each dose over 1 h) according to indication[SPC/BNF] (100 mg bd po for 3 days for cystitis).
☠Stop if tendinitis, severe neuro-Ψ fx or hypersensitivity☠

CITALOPRAM/CIPRAMIL

SSRI antidepressant.
Use: depression[1] (and panic disorder). Useful if polypharmacy, as ↓interactions and ↓cardio-/hepato-toxicity cf other SSRIs.

CI/Caution/SE/Warn: as fluoxetine.
Interactions: ☠*Never give with MAOIs.*☠
Dose: 20 mg od[1] (↑ing if necessary to max 60 mg).

CITRAMAG see Bowel preparations
Dose: 1 sachet at 8am and 3pm the day before GI surgery or Ix.

CLARITHROMYCIN
Macrolide antibiotic: binds 50S ribosome; 'static' at low doses, 'cidal' at high doses.
Use: atypical pneumonias (as alternative to erythromycin; see p. 141), part of triple therapy for *H. pylori* (see p. 145).
CI/Caution/SE/Interactions: as erythromycin, but ⇒ ↓GI SEs.
Dose: 250–500 mg bd po or 500 mg bd iv.

CLEXANE see Enoxaparin; low molecular weight heparin

CLINDAMYCIN
Antibiotic; same action (but different structure and ∴ class) as clarithromycin; good against staphylococci (esp if resistant to penicillin) and anaerobes (esp bacteroides); penetrates bone well.
Use: osteomyelitis, intra-abdominal sepsis, endocarditis Px. Use limited due to SEs, esp AAC.
CI: diarrhoea.
Caution: GI disease, porphyria, atopy, L/R/P/B.
SE: GI upset (often ⇒ **AAC**), hepatotoxicity, blood disorders, local reactions at injection site, hypersensitivity.
Monitor: U&Es, LFTs.
Interactions: ↑s fx of neuromuscular blocking agents.
Dose: 150–450 mg qds po; 0.6–4.8 g daily in divided doses im/ivi (doses >600 mg must be as ivi), max single dose iv is 1.2 g.

Stop drug if diarrhoea develops: AAC common and potentially fatal.

CLOBETASOL PROPIONATE 0.05% CREAM
(DERMOVATE) Very-potent-strength topical corticosteroid.

CLOBETASONE BUTYRATE 0.05% CREAM
(EUMOVATE) Moderately-potent-strength topical corticosteroid.

CLONAZEPAM
Benzodiazepine; long acting (see p. 190)
Use: epilepsy (inc status epilepticus[1]), myoclonus[2]. Not licensed, but often used, for ψ disorders[3] (esp psychosis and mania).
CI/Caution/SE/Warn/Interactions: see Diazepam.
Dose: 1 mg iv (over ⩾2 min) or as ivi[1], repeating if required; 0.5 mg bd ↑ing according to response to max 20 mg/day[2/3].

CLOPIDOGREL/PLAVIX
Antiplatelet agent: ADP receptor antagonist. ↑antiplatelet fx cf aspirin (but also ↑SEs).
Use: Px of atherothrombotic events if NSTEMI (in combination with aspirin), MI (within 'a few' to 35 days), ischaemic CVA (within 7 days to 6 months) or PVD. Now widely used in all ACS (see p. 196).
CI: active bleeding, L (if severe – otherwise caution), **B**.
Caution: ↑bleeding risk; trauma, surgery, drugs that ↑bleeding risk (*not recommended with **warfarin***), R/P.
SE: haemorrhage (esp GI or intracranial), **GI upset**, PU, headache, fatigue, dizziness, paraesthesia, rash/pruritus, hepatobiliary/respiratory/blood disorders (inc, very rarely, TTP).
Monitor: FBC and for signs of occult bleeding (esp after invasive procedures).
Dose: 75 mg od. If not already on clopidogrel, usually load with 300 mg for ACS then 75 mg od starting next day. If pre-PCI, load with 300 mg usually on morning of procedure.
Stop 7 days before operations if antiplatelet fx not wanted (e.g. major surgery); discuss with surgeons doing operation.

L/R/H = Liver, Renal and Heart failure (full key see p. viii)

CLOTRIMAZOLE/CANESTEN
Imidazole antifungal (topical).
Use: external candida infections (esp vaginal thrush).
Caution: can damage condoms and diaphragms.
Dose: 2–3 applications/day of 1% cream, continuing for 14 days after lesion healed. Also available as powder/solution/spray for hairy areas, as pessary, and in 2% strength.

CLOZAPINE
Atypical antipsychotic: blocks dopamine ($D_4 > D_1 > D_{2\&3}$) and $5HT_{2A}$ receptors. Also mild blockade of muscarinic and adrenergic receptors.
Use: schizophrenia, but only if resistant or intolerant (e.g. severe extrapyramidal fx) to other antipsychotics[NICE].
CI: severe cardiac disorders (inc Hx of circulatory collapse, myocarditis, cardiomyopathy, coma/severe CNS depression, alcoholic/toxic psychosis, drug intoxication, Hx of agranulocytosis or ↓NØ, bone marrow disorders, paralytic ileus, uncontrolled epilepsy, **R/H** (if severe, otherwise caution), **L** (inc active liver disease), **B**.
Caution: Hx of epilepsy, cardiovascular disease, ↑prostate, glaucoma (angle-closure), P/E.
SE: as olanzapine, but also can ⇒ ↓NØ (3% of patients) and ☠**agranulocytosis**☠ (1%). Also commonly ⇒ ↑**salivation** (Rx with hyoscine hydrobromide), ↓**BP** (esp during initial titration), **constipation** (can ⇒ ileus/obstruction: have low threshold for giving laxatives), ↑Wt, sedation. Less commonly seizures, urinary incontinence, **myocarditis/cardiomyopathy** (*stop immediately!*), ↑HR, arrhythmias, hyperglycaemia, N&V, ↑BP, delirium. Rarely hepatic dysfunction (*stop immediately!*), ↑TG, neuroleptic malignant syndrome.
Monitor: FBC*, BP (esp during start of Rx), serum levels* (pre-dose) and cardiac function (esp watch for persistent ↑HR).
Interactions: as chlorpromazine, plus care with all drugs that constipate, ↑QT threshold or ↓leukopoiesis (e.g. cytotoxics,

sulphonamides/cotrimoxazole, chloramphenicol, penicillamine, carbamazepine, phenothiazines, esp depots). Caffeine, risperidone, SSRIs, cimetidine and erythromycin ↑clozapine levels. Smoking, carbamazepine and phenytoin ↓clozapine levels.

Dose: initially 12.5 mg nocte, ↑ing to 200–450 mg /day[SPC/BNF] usually given bd (max 900 mg/day).

If >2 days' doses missed, restart at 12.5 mg od and ↑gradually.

> **Monitoring:** primarily to avoid fatal agranulocytosis, is done by the manufacturers: in the UK = Clozaril Patient Monitoring Service (tel: 0845 7698269), Denzapine Monitoring Service (tel: 0845 0090110) or Zaponex Treatment Access System (tel: 0207 3655642) register and then authorise/monitor baseline and subsequent FBCs* and serum levels*.
> *These are very useful resources for all clozapine questions.*

CO-AMILOFRUSE

Diuretic combination preparation for oedema that keeps K^+ stable: amiloride (K^+-sparing) + furosemide (K^+-wasting) in 3 strengths of tablet as 2.5/20, 5/40 and 10/80 (reflecting amiloride mg/furosemide mg).

Dose: 1 tablet mane (NB: *specify strength!*).

CO-AMILOZIDE

Diuretic combination preparation for HTN, CCF and oedema. Keeps K^+ stable: amiloride (K^+-sparing) + hydrochlorothiazide (K^+-wasting) in 2 strengths of tablet as 2.5/25 and 5/50 (reflecting amiloride mg/hydrochlorothiazide mg).

Dose: 1/2–4 tablets daily, according to tablet strength and indication[SPC/BNF].

CO-AMOXICLAV/AUGMENTIN

Combination of amoxicillin + clavulanic acid (β-lactamase inhibitor) to overcome resistance.

L/R/H = **L**iver, **R**enal and **H**eart failure (full key see p. viii)

Use: UTIs, respiratory/skin/soft-tissue (plus many other) infections. Reserve for when β-lactamase-producing strains known/strongly suspected or other Rx has failed.
Cl/Caution/SE/Interactions: as ampicillin, plus caution if anticoagulated, **L** (↑risk of cholestasis), **P**.
Dose: 375 or 625 mg tds po; 1.2 g tds iv (= combined dose of the 2 drugs). Non-proprietary and as Augmentin.

CO-BENELDOPA/MADOPAR

L-dopa + benserazide (peripheral dopa-decarboxylase inhibitor).
Use: parkinsonism.
Cl/Caution/SE/Warn/Interactions: see Levodopa.
Dose: (*expressed as levodopa only*) initially 50 mg tds/qds, ↑ing total dose and number of doses, according to response, to usual maintenance of 400–800 mg/day (↓ in elderly).

CO-CARELDOPA/SINEMET

L-dopa + carbidopa (peripheral dopa-decarboxylase inhibitor).
Use: parkinsonism.
Cl/Caution/SE/Warn/Interactions: see Levodopa.
Dose: (*expressed as levodopa only*) initially 50–100 mg tds, ↑ing total dose and number of doses, according to response, to usual maintenance of 400–800 mg/day (↓ in elderly).

CO-CODAMOL (8/500) = codeine 8 mg + paracetamol 500 mg
per tablet. Dose: 2 tablets qds prn.

CO-DANTHRAMER see Dantron; stimulant laxative.
Dose: 1–2 capsules or 5–10 ml suspension nocte (available in regular and strong formulations).

CO-DANTHRUSATE see Dantron; stimulant laxative.
Dose: 1–3 capsules or 5–15 ml suspension nocte.

CODEINE (PHOSPHATE)

Opioid analgesic.

Use: mild/moderate pain, diarrhoea, cough (as linctus).

CI/Caution/SE/Interactions: as morphine, but milder SEs
(**constipation** is the major problem: dose and length of Rx-dependent;
anticipate this and give laxative Px as appropriate, esp in elderly).

Dose: 30–60 mg up to qds po/im.

CO-DYDRAMOL = dihydrocodeine 10 mg + paracetamol
500 mg per tablet. Dose: 2 tablets qds po prn.

COLCHICINE

Anti-gout: binds to tubulin of leukocytes and stops their migration
to uric acid deposits ∴ ⇒ ↓inflammation. NB: slow action
(needs >6 h to work).

Use: gout: Rx of acute attacks or Px when starting allopurinol*
(which can initially ↑symptoms) or awaiting other drugs to work.

CI: blood dyscrasias, **P**

Caution: GI diseases, L/H/R/B/E.

SE: GI upset (N&V&D and **abdominal pain** – all common and
dose-related). Rarely GI haemorrhage, hypersensitivity, renal/hepatic
impairment, peripheral neuritis, myopathy, alopecia,
↓spermatogenesis (reversible), blood disorders (if prolonged Rx).

Interactions: ↑s nephro-/myo-toxicity of ciclosporin, fx ↓by
thiazide diuretics, toxicity ↑by erythromycin and tolbutamide.

Dose: 0.5 mg tds for 7 days (start ASAP after symptom onset).
More aggressive loading regimens exist[SPC/BNF] but ⇒ ↑GI upset w/o
significant ↑ in response. Continue 0.5 mg tds for 3 months when
starting allopurinol*.

CORSODYL Chlorhexidine mouthwash for Rx/Px of mouth
infections (inc MRSA eradication); see local infection protocol.

CO-TRIAMTERZIDE

Diuretic for HTN[1] or oedema[2]: triamterene (↑s K$^+$) combined with
hydrochlorothiazide (↓s K$^+$) to keep K$^+$ stable.

L/R/H = **L**iver, **R**enal and **H**eart failure (full key see p. viii)

Dose: initially 1 tablet[1] (or 2 tablets[2]) mane of 50/25 strength (= 50 mg triamterene + 25 mg hydrochlorothiazide), ↑ing if necessary to max of 4 tablets/day.

CO-TRIMOXAZOLE/SEPTRIN

Antibiotic combination preparation: 5 to 1 mixture of sulfamethoxazole (a sulphonamide) + trimethoprim ⇒ synergistic action (individually are 'static' but collectively are 'cidal').
Use: PCP; other uses limited due to SEs (also rarely used for toxoplasmosis and nocardiasis).
CI: porphyria, **L/R** (if either severe, otherwise caution).
Caution: blood disorders, asthma, G6PD deficiency, P/B/E.
SE: skin reactions (inc SJS, TEN), **blood disorders** (↓NØ, ↓Pt, BM suppression, agranulocytosis) relatively common, esp in elderly. Also N&V&D (inc AAC), nephrotoxicity, hepatotoxicity, hypersensitivity, anorexia, abdominal pain, glossitis, stomatitis, pancreatitis, arthralgia, myalgia, SLE, pulmonary infiltrates, seizures.
Interactions: ↑s phenytoin levels. ↑s risk of arrhythmias with amiodarone, crystalluria with methenamine, antifolate fx with pyrimethamine, agranulocytosis with clozapine and toxicity with ciclosporin, azathioprine, mercaptopurine and methotrexate. **W+**.
Dose: PCP Rx: 120 mg/kg/day po/ivi in 2–4 divided doses (PCP Px 480–960 mg od po).

☠ Stop immediately if rash or blood disorder occurs. ☠

CYCLIZINE

Antihistamine antiemetic.
Use: N&V Rx/Px (esp 2° to iv/im opioids, but not 1st choice in angina/MI/LVF*), vertigo, motion sickness, labyrinthine disorders.
CI/Caution/SE/Warn: as chlorphenamine, but also avoid in severe HF* (may undo haemodynamic benefits of opioids). Antimuscarinic fx (see p. 191) are most prominent SEs.
Dose: 50 mg po/im/iv tds.

CYCLOPHOSPHAMIDE

Cytotoxic[1] and immunosuppressant[2]: alkylating agent (cross-links DNA bases, ↓ing replication).

Use: Cancer[1], autoimmune diseases[2]: esp vasculitis (inc rheumatoid arthritis, polymyositis and SLE (esp if renal/cerebral involvement)), systemic sclerosis, Wegener's, nephrotic syndrome in children.

CI: haemorrhagic cystitis **P/B**.

Caution: BM suppression, severe infections, **L/R**.

SE: GI upset, alopecia (reversible). Others rare but important: hepatotoxicity, blood disorders, malignancy (esp acute non-lymphocytic leukaemia), ↓fertility (can be permanent), pulmonary fibrosis (at high doses), haemorrhagic cystitis (only if given iv: ensure good hydration, give 'mesna' as Px; can occur months after Rx).

Warn: ↓fertility may be permanent (bank sperm if possible) – need to counsel and obtain consent regarding this before giving.

Monitor: FBC.

Interactions: can ↑fx of oral hypoglycaemics. ↑risk of agranulocytosis with clozapine and toxicity with pentostatin.

Dose: specialist use only.

☠ Stop immediately if rash or blood disorder occurs. ☠

CYCLOSPORIN see Ciclosporin

CYPROTERONE ACETATE

Anti-androgen; blocks androgen receptors. Also ↑s progestogens.

Use: Ca prostate[1] (as adjunct), acne[2] (esp 2° to PCOS, where used with ethinylestradiol as co-cyprindiol), rarely for hypersexuality/sexual deviation[3] (*males only!*).

CI: (*none apply if for Ca prostate*) advanced DM (if vascular disease), sickle cell, malignancy/wasting diseases, Hx of TE, age <18 years (can ⇒ bone/testicular development), severe depression, **L/P/B**.

SE: fatigue, gynaecomastia, ↑ or ↓Wt, hepatotoxicity, blood disorders, hypersensitivity, osteoporosis, ↓spermatogenesis (reversible), TE, depression, carbohydrate metabolism and hair Δs.

Monitor: FBC, LFTs, adrenocortical function.
Warn: driving and other skilled tasks may be impaired.
Dose: 200–300 mg po daily in divided doses[1], 50 mg bd po[3].

DALTEPARIN/FRAGMIN

Low-molecular-weight heparin (LMWH).
Use: DVT/PE Rx[1] and Px[2] (inc preoperative), ACS (with aspirin)[3].
CI/Caution/SE/Monitor/Interactions: see Heparin.
Dose: *all sc:* 200 units/kg (max 18 000 units) od[1]; 2500–5000 units od[2] (according to risk[SPC/BNF]) for ⩾5 days; 120 units/kg bd[3] for ⩾ 5 days (max 10 000 units bd) reviewing dose if >8 days needed [SPC/BNF].
Consider monitoring anti Xa (3–4 h post dose) if RF (i.e. creatinine >150), pregnancy, Wt >100 kg or <45 kg; see p. 175.

DANTRON

Stimulant laxative; theoretical risk of **cardiogenicity***.
Use: constipation (often limited to the terminally ill*)
Caution/SE: see Senna. (☠ CI if GI obstruction, **P/B** ☠)
Dose: see Co-danthramer and Co-danthrusate.

▼DARBEPOETIN see Erythropoietin (recombinant form for ↓Hb)

DERMOVATE see Clobetasol propionate (steroid) cream 0.05%

DESFERRIOXAMINE

Chelating agent; binds Fe (and Al) in gut ↓ing absorption.
Use: ↑Fe: acute (OD/poisoning[1]), chronic (e.g. xs transfusions for blood disorders, haemochromatosis when venesection CI). Also for ↑Al (e.g. 2° to dialysis).
Caution: Al-induced encephalopathy (may worsen), R/P/B.
SE: ↓BP (related to rate of ivi), lens opacities, retinopathy, GI upset, blood disorders, hypersensitivity. Also neurological/respiratory/renal dysfunction. ↑doses can ⇒ ↓growth and bone Δs.
Monitor: vision and hearing during chronic Rx.

Dose: acutely up to 15 mg/kg/h ivi (max 80 mg/kg/day)[1]. Otherwise according to degree of Fe or Al overload[SPC/BNF].

DEXAMETHASONE PHOSPHATE

Glucocorticoid; minimal mineralocorticoid activity, long duration of action (see p. 185).

Use: cerebral oedema, Dx of Cushing's, N&V (2° to chemotherapy or surgery), allergy/inflammation (esp if unresponsive shock), congenital adrenal hyperplasia.

CI/Caution/SE/Warn/Interactions: see Prednisolone and steroids section (pp. 185–7).

Dose: cerebral oedema: acutely 10 mg iv, then 4 mg im qds (if not life-threatening, some go straight to 4 mg qds iv then switch to po a few days later). For other indications, see SPC/BNF.

☠Doses given here are for *dexamethasone phosphate* and must be prescribed as such: other forms have different doses!☠

DF118 (suffix FORTE often omitted) Dihydrocodeine preparation.
Dose: 40–80 mg tds po (max 240 mg/day); 50 mg sc/im 4–6 hourly.
NB: tablets are different dose to non-proprietary dihydrocodeine.

DIAMORPHINE

Strong opioid (1.5 × strength of morphine if both given iv): analgesic, anxiolytic and beneficial cardiac fx*: ↓s myocardial O_2 demand and ⇒ transient venodilation (↓s preload, cardiac filling pressures and pulmonary congestion).

Use: severe pain[1]. Also acute MI[2], ACS[2] or acute pulmonary oedema*[2].

CI/Caution/SE/Interactions: as Morphine, but less nausea/↓BP.
☠**Respiratory depression** (esp elderly) and **constipation**☠.

Dose: 5–10 mg sc/im (or 1/4–1/2 this dose iv) up to 4-hourly[1]; 2.5–5 mg iv (at 1 mg/min)[2]. Can give as sc pump in chronic pain/palliative care; see pp. 156–8.

DIAZEMULS iv diazepam *emulsion*: ⇒ ↓venous irritation.

DIAZEPAM

Benzodiazepine, long-acting.

Use: seizures (esp status epilepticus[1], febrile convulsions), *short-term* Rx of acute alcohol withdrawal[2], anxiety[3], insomnia[4] (if also anxiety; if not, then shorter-acting forms preferred as ⇒ ↓hangover sedation). Also used for muscle spasm[5].

CI: respiratory depression, sleep apnoea, acute pulmonary insufficiency, chronic psychosis, depression (if diazepam given alone), phobic/obsessional states, **L** (if severe).

Caution: respiratory disease, muscle weakness (inc MG), Hx of drug/alcohol abuse, personality disorder, porphyria, R/P/B/E.

SE: respiratory depression, drowsiness, dependence. Also ataxia, amnesia, headache, vertigo, GI upset, jaundice, ↓BP, ↓HR, visual/libido/urinary disturbances.

Warn: sedation ↑by alcohol and ⇒ ↓driving/skilled task ability.

Interactions: metab by **P450** ∴ many but most importantly: sedative fx ↑by antipsychotics, antidepressants, antiepileptics and antiretrovirals. Ery-/clari-thromycin and flu-/itra-/keto-conazole can ↑levels. Can ↑zidovudine levels.

Dose: for status epilepticus[1] and alcohol withdrawal[2], see pp. 203 and 161, respectively; 2 mg tds po (↑ up to 30 mg/day)[3,5]; 5–15 mg nocte po[4]. ↓dose if elderly or LF. If chronic exposure to benzodiazepines, ↑doses may be needed; do not stop suddenly, as can ⇒ withdrawal; see p. 189 for details.

> 🐝 **Respiratory depression:** if ↑doses used (esp iv/im), monitor O_2 sats and have flumazenil and O_2 (± intubation equipment) at hand — see pp. 215–16 for Mx 🐝

DICLOFENAC

Medium-strength NSAID; non-selective COX inhibitor.

Use: pain/inflammation, esp musculoskeletal; rheumatoid arthritis, osteoarthritis, acute gout, postoperative (esp orthopaedic).

CI/Caution/SE/Interactions: as Ibuprofen, plus avoid in porphyria (↓risk of GI ulcer/bleeds if given with misoprostol as Arthrotec).

Dose: 50 mg tds po or 75 mg bd po (or im, but for max of 2 days); (12.5–) 100 mg pr. Max 150 mg/day. Rarely used iv[BNF/SPC].

DIDRONEL PMO see Etidronate; osteoporosis Rx/Px.

DIFFLAM Benzydamine: topical NSAID.
Use: mouth ulcers, radio-/chemo-therapy-induced mucositis as spray
(4–8 sprays 1.5–3-hourly) or oral rinse (15 ml 1.5–3-hourly).
Available as cream for musculoskeletal pain.

DIGIBIND Anti-digoxin Ab for digoxin toxicity/OD unresponsive
to supportive Rx. See SPC for dose.

DIGOXIN

Cardiac glycoside: ↓s HR by slowing AVN conduction and ↑ing
vagal tone. Also weak inotrope.
Use: AF (and other SVTs), HF.
CI: HB (intermittent complete), 2nd-degree AV block, VF, VT,
HOCM (can use with care if also AF and HF), SVTs 2° to WPW.
Caution: recent MI, ↓K^+*/↓T_4 (both ⇒ ↑digoxin toxicity*), SSS,
rhythms resembling AF (e.g. atrial tachycardia with variable AV
block), R/E (↓dose), P.
SE: generally mild unless rapid ivi, xs Rx or OD: **GI upset** (esp
nausea), **arrhythmias/HB, neuro-Ψ disturbances** (inc visual Δs,
esp blurred vision and yellow/green halos), fatigue, weakness,
confusion, hallucinations, mood Δs. Also gynaecomastia (if chronic
Rx), rarely ↓Pt, rash.
Monitor: U&Es, digoxin levels (ideally take 6 h post-dose:
therapeutic range = 1–2 µg/l).
Interactions: digoxin fx/toxicity ↑d by Ca^{2+} antagonists (esp
verapamil), amiodarone, propafenone, quinidine, antimalarials,
itraconazole, amphotericin, ciclosporin, St John's wort and diuretics
(mostly via ↓K^+*), but also ACE-i/ARBs and spironolactone (despite
potential ↑K^+). Cholestyramine and antacids can ↓ digoxin absorption.
Dose: *non-acute:* load with 125–250 µg bd po (maintenance dose
62.5–375 µg od). ↓dose if RF, elderly or digoxin given <2 wks ago.

Digoxin loading for acute AF: *either* 0.75–1 mg as ivi over 2 h *or*
500 µg po repeated 12 h later. Then follow non-acute schedule.

DIHYDROCODEINE see Codeine; similar-strength opioid.
Dose: 30–60 mg up to qds po (or up to 50 mg qds im/sc) with or after food. ↑doses can be given under close supervision.

DILATING EYE DROPS for fundoscopy:

1 **Tropicamide 1%** Most common; CI if Hx of angle-closure glaucoma (cloudy cornea should raise suspicion) but OK if open-angle/simple glaucoma.
2 **Phenylephrine 2.5% or 10%** Better for Asian and black patients, as ↓ response to tropicamide is common. CI if angle closure glaucoma and avoid if limbal ischaemia (e.g. after chemical injury). Also CI if cardiac disease, HTN, ↑HR, aneurysms, ↑T_4, longstanding DM and if on MAOI, TCA or antihypertensive.

Consider cycloplegic forms (e.g. cyclopentolate) for children or if corneal abrasions, as they are more comfortable for examination.

DILTIAZEM

Rate-limiting benzothiazepine Ca^{2+} channel blocker: ↓s HR and contractility* (but <verapamil) and ↓s BP. Also dilates peripheral/coronary arteries.
Use: Rx/Px of angina[1] (esp if β-blockers CI) and HTN[2].
CI: LVF* with pulmonary congestion, ↓↓HR, 2nd/3rd-degree AV block (without pacemaker), SSS, **P/B**.
Caution: 1st-degree AV block, ↓HR, ↑PR interval, L/R/H.
SE: headache, flushing, GI upset (esp **N&C**), **oedema** (esp ankle), ↓HR, ↓BP. Rarely SAN/AVN block, arrhythmias, rash, hepatotoxicity.
Interactions: β-blockers and verapamil (can ⇒ asystole, AV block, ↓↓HR, HF). ↑s fx of digoxin, ciclosporin, theophyllines, carbamazepine and phenytoin. ☠️↑risk of VF with iv dandrolene.☠️
Dose: 60 mg tds (↑ing to max of 360 mg/day)[1]; 180–480 mg/day in 1 or 2 doses[2] (*suitable for HTN only as MR preparation: no non-proprietary forms exist and brands vary in clinical fx ∴ specify which is required*[SPC/BNF]). Consider ↓ing doses if LF or RF.

DIPROBASE Paraffin-based emollient cream/ointment for dry skin conditions (e.g. eczema, psoriasis).

DIPYRIDAMOLE/PERSANTIN

Antiplatelet agent: inhibits Pt aggregation, adhesion and survival (also $\Rightarrow$ arterial dilation: inc coronaries).

Use: 2° prevention of ischaemic TIA/CVA[1], Px of TE from prosthetic valves (as adjunct to warfarin)[2].

Caution: recent MI, angina (if unstable), aortic stenosis, coagulation disorders, ↓BP, MG*, migraine (may worsen), H.

SE: GI upset, dizziness, myalgia, headache, ↓BP, ↑HR, hot flushes, rarely worsening of IHD, hypersensitivity (rash, urticaria, bronchospasm, angioedema), ↑postoperative bleeding, ↓Pt.

Interactions: ↓s fx (but ↑s hypotensive fx) of cholinesterase inhibitors*, ↑s fx of adenosine. **W+**.

Dose: 200 mg bd po as MR preparation (Persantin retard)[1,2]; 100–200 mg tds po[2]. All doses to be taken with food.

DISULFIRAM/ANTABUSE

Alcohol dehydrogenase inhibitor: $\Rightarrow$ ↑systemic acetaldehyde $\Rightarrow$ unpleasant SE when alcohol ingested (inc small amounts ∴ care with alcohol-containing medications, foods, toiletries).

Use: alcohol withdrawal (maintenance of).

CI: Hx of IHD or CVA, HTN, psychosis, ↑suicide risk, severe personality disorder, **H/P/B**.

Caution: DM, epilepsy, respiratory disease, **L/R**.

SE: only if alcohol ingested – N&V, flushing, headache, ↑HR, ↓BP (± collapse if xs alcohol intake).

Interactions: ↑s fx of phenytoin, ↑toxicity with paraldehyde **W+**.

Dose: initially 800 mg od, ↓ing to 100–200 mg od over 5 days.

NB: Must have consumed no alcohol within at least 24 h of 1st dose.

DOBUTAMINE

Inotropic sympathomimetic: mostly β_1 fx $\Rightarrow$ ↑contractility. ↓fx on HR compared with dopamine.

Use: shock (cardiogenic, septic).
Caution: severe ↓BP.
SE: ↑HR, ↑BP (if xs Rx).
Interactions: risk of ↑BP crisis with β-blockers (esp if 'non-selective').
Dose: 2.5–10 μg/kg/min ivi, titrating to response (via central line, preferably with invasive cardiac monitoring). Often given with dopamine; seek expert help.

DOCUSATE SODIUM

Stimulant laxative: ⇒ ↑GI motility (also a softening agent).
Use/Caution/SE: see Senna (☠ **CI if GI obstruction** ☠).
Dose: 50–100 mg up to tds po (max 500 mg/day). Also available as enemas[SPC/BNF].

DOMPERIDONE

Antiemetic: D$_2$ antagonist – inhibits central nausea chemoreceptor trigger zone. Poor BBB penetration ∴ ↓central SEs (extrapyramidal fx, sedation) cf other dopamine antagonists.
Use: N&V, esp 2° to chemotherapy or 'morning-after pill', and in Parkinson's disease or migraine. Rarely for gastro-oesophageal reflux and dyspepsia.
CI: prolactinoma, when GI obstruction harmful, **L**.
Caution: GI obstruction **R/P/B**.
SE: rash, allergy, ↑prolactin (can ⇒ gynaecomastia and galactorrhoea). Rarely ↓libido, dystonia and extrapyramidal fx.
Dose: 10 mg tds po (can ↑ to max 20 mg qds); 60 mg bd pr. Not available im/iv.

DONEPEZIL/ARICEPT

Acetylcholinesterase inhibitor (reversible); see Rivastigmine.
Use: Alzheimer's disease[NICE].
CI: P/B.
Caution: supraventricular conduction dfx (esp SSS), ↑risk of PU (e.g. Hx of PU or NSAID), COPD/asthma, extrapyramidal symptoms can worsen, **L**.

SE: cholinergic fx (see p. 191), **GI upset** (esp initially), **insomnia** (if occurs, change dose to mane), **headache**, fatigue, dizziness, syncope, rash, Ψ disturbances. Rarely ↓ or ↑BP, seizures, PU/GI bleeds, SAN/AVN block, hepatotoxicity.

Interactions: metab by **P450** ∴ inhibitors and inducers on p. 193 could ↑or ↓levels, respectively; check BNF/SPC.

Dose: 5 mg nocte (↑ to 10 mg after 1 month if necessary); specialist use only – need review for clinical response and tolerance.

DOPAMINE

Inotropic sympathomimetic: dose-dependent fx on receptors: low doses (2–3 µg/kg/min) stimulate peripheral DA receptors but little else ∴ ⇒ ↑renal perfusion*; higher doses (>5 µg/kg/min) also have β_1 fx (⇒ ↑ contractility); even higher doses have α fx (⇒ vaso-constriction, but can worsen HF).

Use: shock, esp if ARF* or cardiogenic (e.g. post-MI or cardiac surgery).

CI: tachyarrhythmias, phaeo, ↑T_4.

Caution: correct hypovolaemia before giving.

SE: N&V, ↓ or ↑BP, ↑HR, peripheral vasoconstriction.

Interactions: fx ↑by cyclopropane and halogen hydrocarbon anaesthetics (are CI) or MAOIs (can ⇒ ↑↑BP; consider ↓↓dose of dopamine).

Dose: initially 2–5 µg/kg/min ivi (via central line, preferably with invasive cardiac monitoring), then adjust to response; seek specialist help.

DORZOLAMIDE/TRUSOPT

Topical carbonic anhydrase inhibitor: as Acetazolamide (oral preparation, which is more potent but has ↑SEs*).

Use: glaucoma (esp if β-blocker CI or fails to ↓IOP).

CI: ↑Cl^- acidosis, **R** (severe only), **P/B**.

Caution: Hx of renal stones† or intraocular surgery, corneal dfx, **L**.

SE: local irritation, blurred vision, bitter taste, anterior uveitis, rash. Rarely* systemic SEs (esp urolithiasis†) and interactions; see Acetazolamide.

Dose: apply 2% drop tds. Available as bd prep with timolol (Cosopt).

DOXAPRAM

Respiratory stimulant: $\uparrow$s activity of respiratory and vasomotor centres in medulla $\Rightarrow$ $\uparrow$depth (and, to lesser extent, rate) of breathing. Also indirect fx by stimulation of chemoreceptors in aorta and carotid artery.

Use: hypoventilation, life-threatening respiratory failure – usually only if dt transient/reversible cause, e.g. post-operative/-general anaesthetic or acute deterioration with known precipitant. Mostly used in preventing respiratory depression $2°$ to $\uparrow FiO_2$ used in severe respiratory acidosis (can be harmful if $CO_2 \downarrow$ or normal).

CI: severe asthma or HTN, IHD, $\uparrow T_4$, epilepsy, physical obstruction of respiratory tract.

Caution: if taking MAOIs, L/H/P.

SE: headache, flushing, chest pains, arrhythmias, vasoconstriction, $\uparrow$BP, $\uparrow$HR, laryngo-/broncho-spasm, GI upset, dizziness, seizures.

Dose: specialist use only (mostly in ITU).

DOXAZOSIN/CARDURA

α_1 blocker $\Rightarrow$ systemic vasodilation and relaxation of internal urethral sphincter $\therefore \Rightarrow \downarrow$TPR[1] and $\uparrow$bladder outflow[2].

Use: HTN[1], BPH[2].

CI: B.

Caution: postural $\downarrow$BP, micturition syncope, L/H/P/E.

SE: postural $\downarrow$BP (esp after 1st dose*), **dizziness, headache, urinary incontinence** (esp women), GI upset (esp N&V), drowsiness/fatigue, syncope, mood Δs, dry mouth, oedema, somnolence, blurred vision, rhinitis. Rarely erectile dysfunction, $\uparrow$HR, arrhythmias, hypersensitivity/rash. Chronic Rx $\Rightarrow$ beneficial lipid Δs ($\uparrow$HDL, $\downarrow$LDL, $\downarrow$VLDL, $\downarrow$TG).

Interactions: $\uparrow$s hypotensive fx of diuretics, β-blockers, Ca^{2+} antagonists, silden-/tadal-/varden-afil, anaesthetics and antidepressants.

Dose: initially 1 mg od (give 1st dose before bed*), then slowly $\uparrow$ according to response (max 16 mg/day[1] or 8 mg/day[2]). 4 or 8 mg od if MR preparation, as Cardura XL.

DOXYCYCLINE

Tetracycline antibiotic: inhibits ribosomal (30S) subunit. Has longest $t_{1/2}$ of all tetracyclines $\therefore$ od dosing.

Use: genital infections, esp syphilis, chlamydia, PID, salpingitis, urethritis (non-gonococcal). Also **tropical diseases**, e.g. rickettsia (inc Q fever), *Brucella*, Lyme disease (*Borrelia burgdorferi*), malaria (Px/Rx, not 1st-line), mycoplasma (genital/respiratory), COPD infective exac (*H. influenzae*), **anthrax** (Rx/Px).

CI/Caution/SE/Interactions: as tetracycline, but can give with caution if RF, although is CI in porphyria, SLE and achlorhydria.

Warn: avoid UV light and Zn-/Fe-containing products (e.g. antacids).

Dose: 100–200 mg od/bd[SPC/BNF].

EDROPHONIUM

Short-acting anticholinesterase given iv/im during Tensilon test for Dx of MG – look for ↓symptoms (i.e. ↑strength).

ENALAPRIL/INNOVACE

ACE-i.

Use/CI/Caution/SE/Interactions: as Captopril, plus L.

Dose: initially 2.5 mg od (5 mg if for HTN and not elderly, on diuretics or RF), then ↑ according to response (max 40 mg od).

ENOXAPARIN/CLEXANE

Low-molecular-weight heparin (LMWH).

Use: DVT/PE Rx[1] and Px[2] (inc preoperative), ACS (with aspirin)[3].

CI/Caution/SE/Monitor/Interactions: as Heparin, plus B.

Dose: (all sc; 1 mg = 100 units) 1.5 mg/kg od[1], 40 mg od (20 mg od if not high risk)[2], 1 mg/kg bd[3].

Consider monitoring anti Xa (3–4 h post dose) if RF (i.e. creatinine >150), pregnancy, Wt >100 kg or <45 kg; see p. 175.

ENSURE Protein and calorie supplement drinks.

L/R/H = Liver, Renal and Heart failure (full key see p. viii)

EPILIM see Valproate

EPINEPHRINE see Adrenaline

EPOETIN see Erythropoietin (recombinant form for ↓Hb).

EPROSARTAN/TEVETEN
Angiotensin II antagonist; see Losartan.
Use: HTN
CI: L (if severe), **P/B**.
Caution/SE/Interactions: see Losartan.
Dose: 600 mg od (max 800 mg od). Start at 300 mg and then ↑ as required if elderly, RF or LF.

EPTIFIBATIDE/INTEGRILIN
Antiplatelet agent: glycoprotein IIb/IIIa receptor inhibitor – stops binding of fibrinogen and inhibits platelet aggregation.
Use: Px of MI in unstable angina and NSTEMI (if last episode of chest pain w/in 24 h), esp if high risk and awaiting PCI[NICE] (see p. 198).
CI: haemorrhagic diathesis, severe trauma or major surgery w/in 6 weeks, abnormal bleeding or CVA w/in 30 days, Hx of haemorrhagic CVA or intracranial disease (AVM, aneurysm or neoplasm), ↓Pt ,↑INR, severe HTN, **L** (if significant), **R** (if severe), **B**.
Caution: drugs that ↑bleeding risk (esp thrombolysis), **P**.
SE: bleeding.
Monitor: FBC (baseline, w/in 6 h of giving, then at least daily) plus clotting and creatinine (baseline at least).
Dose: initially 180 µg/kg iv bolus followed by ivi of 2 µg/kg/min for up to 72 h (or 96 h if awaiting PCI). Needs concurrent heparin. Specialist use only: get senior advice or contact on-call cardiology.

ERGOCALCIFEROL (= CALCIFEROL)
Vit D_2: needs renal (1) and hepatic (25) hydroxylation for activation.

Use: vitamin D deficiency.

CI: ↑Ca^{2+}, metastatic calcification.

Caution: R (if high 'pharmacological'* doses used), B.

SE: ↑Ca^{2+}. If over-Rx: **GI upset**, weakness, headache, polydipsia/polyuria, anorexia, RF, arrhythmias.

Monitor: Ca^{2+} (esp if N&V develops or ↑doses in RF*).

Interactions: fx ↓by anticonvulsants and ↑by thiazides.

Dose: 10–20 μg (400–800 units) od as part of multivitamin preparations or combined with calcium lactate or phosphate as 'calcium + ergocalciferol': non-proprietary preparations available but is often prescribed by trade name (e.g. Cacit D3, or Calcichew D3). ↑doses of 0.25–1.0 mg od (of 'pharmacological strength' preparations*) used for GI malabsorption and chronic liver disease (up to 5 mg daily for ↓PTH or renal osteodystrophy).

*Specify strength of tablet required to avoid confusion[SPC/BNF].

ERYTHROMYCIN

Macrolide antibiotic: binds 50S ribosome; 'static' at low doses, 'cidal' at high doses.

Use: atypical pneumonias (with other agents; see p. 141), rarely *Chlamydia*/other GU infections, *Campylobacter enteritis*. Often used if allergy to penicillin.

CI: macrolide hypersensitivity or if taking terfenadine, pimozide, ergotamine or dihydroergotamine.

Caution: ↑QTc (inc drugs that predispose to), porphyria, L/R/P/B.

SE: GI upset (rarely AAC), **dry itchy skin**, hypersensitivity (inc SJS, TEN), arrhythmias (esp VT), chest pain, reversible hearing loss (dose-related, esp if RF), cholestatic jaundice.

Interactions: ↓P450 ∴ many; most importantly ↑s levels of ciclosporin, digoxin, theophyllines and carbamazepine, **W+**.

Dose: 500 mg qds po (250 mg qds if mild infection, 1 g qds if severe); 50 mg/kg daily iv in 4 divided doses.

NB: venous irritant ∴ give po if possible.

ERYTHROPOIETIN

Recombinant erythropoietin.

Use: ↓Hb 2° to CRF or chemotherapy (AZT or platinum-containing). Also unlicensed use for myeloma, lymphoma and certain myelodysplasias. 3 types: α (Eprex), β (NeoRecormon) and longer-acting darbepoetin (▼Aranesp).

SE: ↑BP, ↑K+, headache, arthralgia, oedema, TE. ☠Rarely ⇒ red cell aplasia (esp subcutaneous Eprex if RF, which if now CI).☠

CI/Caution/Dose: specialist use only^SPC/BNF; given subcutaneously (self-administered) or iv (as inpatient). ↓Fe/folate (monitor), ↑Al, infections and inflammatory disease can ↓response.

ESMOLOL

β-blocker: cardioselective ($β_1 > β_2$) and short-acting*.

Use: SVTs (inc AF, atrial flutter, sinus ↑HR), HTN (esp perioperatively), acute MI (*safer than long-acting preparations).

CI/Caution/SE/Interactions: see Propranolol.

Dose: usually 50–200 μg/kg/min ivi, preceded by loading dose if perioperative^SPC.

ESOMEPRAZOLE/NEXIUM

PPI; as Omeprazole, plus **R**.

Dose: 20 mg od po (40 mg od for 1st 4 wks, if for gastro-oesophageal reflux); 20–40 mg/day iv^SPC/BNF (▼).

ETANERCEPT/ENBREL

Monoclonal Ab against TNF-α (an inflammatory cytokine).

Use: severe arthritis (rheumatoid^NICE, juvenile idiopathic^NICE and psoriatic), severe plaque psoriasis and ankylosing spondylitis.

CI/Caution/Interactions: See SPC.

SE: blood disorders, severe infections, CNS demyelination, GI upset, exac of HF, headache. *Specialist use only.*

☠Do not give live vaccines during Rx.☠

ETHAMBUTOL

Anti-TB antibiotic: inhibits cell-wall synthesis ('static').

Use: TB initial Rx phase (1st 2 months) *if isoniazid resistance known or suspected* (see pp. 145–6).

CI: optic neuritis, ↓vision.

Caution: R (monitor levels* and ↓dose if creatinine clearance <30 ml/min), P/E.

SE: neuritis; peripheral and **optic** (can ⇒ ↓visual acuity**, colour-blindness, ↓visual fields ∴ ⇒ baseline and regular ophthalmology review). Rarely GI upset, skin reactions, ↓Pt.

Warn: patient to report immediately any visual symptoms – use alternative drug if unable to do this (e.g. very young, ↓IQ).

Monitor: visual acuity** (inc baseline before Rx), plasma levels*.

Dose: 15 mg/kg od (30 mg/kg 3 times a week if 'supervised' Rx).

(DISODIUM) ETIDRONATE

Bisphosphonate: ↓s bone turnover.

Use: osteoporosis Rx/Px[1] (if alendronate or risedronate not suitable/tolerated), Paget's disease[2].

CI: ↑Ca^{2+} (in blood or urine), clinically overt osteomalacia, R (caution only if mild; ↓dose), P/B.

SE: GI upset, ↑PO_4 (transient *NB: other bisphosphonates ↓PO_4!*). Can ⇒ bone pain in Paget's disease (stop if ⇒ fractures). Rarely, neurological disorders (headache, paraesthesia, peripheral neuropathy), blood disorders, hypersensitivity/skin reactions.

Monitor: ALP, Ca^{2+}, PO_4 (and urinary hydroxyproline[2]).

Warn: avoid food for ≥2 h after taking, esp Ca^{2+}-containing products (milk, Fe/mineral supplements, antacids).

Dose: 400 mg for 14 days followed by 1.25 g $CaCO_3$ for 76 days (as Didronel PMO in 90-day packs: 1 tablet od)[1]; 5–20 mg/kg/day po[2].

ETODOLAC

Medium-strength NSAID, selective COX2 inhibitor; but not as selective as cele-/etori-coxib, which ⇒ ↑cardiovascular risk.

Use: osteo- or rheumatoid arthritis symptom relief[NICE].

CI/Caution/SE/Interactions: see Ibuprofen.
Dose: 300 mg bd (or 600 mg od as Lodine SR).

▼**ETORICOXIB/**ARCOXIA
NSAID, selective COX2 inhibitor.
Use: osteo[1]/rheumatoid[2] arthritis[NICE], acute gout[3].
CI/Caution/SE/Interactions: as Celecoxib, plus CI in
uncontrolled HTN.
Dose: 60 mg od[1]; 90 mg od[2]; 120 mg od[3].

EUMOVATE see Clobetasone butyrate 0.05%; steroid cream.

FANSIDAR
Antimalarial: combination tablet of pyrimethamine (25 mg) +
sulfadoxine (500 mg).
Use: Rx of falciparum malaria (with or following quinine).
CI: sulphonamide or pyrimethamine allergy, porphyria
Caution: blood disorders, asthma, G6PD deficiency, L/R/P/B/E.
SE: blood disorders, skin reactions*, pulmonary infiltrates,
insomnia, GI upset, nephrotoxicity, hepatotoxicity, hypersensitivity.
Monitor: FBC (if chronic Rx) and for rash* or cough/SOB (stop drug).
Dose: see pp. 145–6.

FENTANYL
Strong opiate; used in palliative care as lozenge (Actiq) or topical
slow-release patch (Durogesic) and in anaesthesia iv.
CI/Caution/SE/Interactions: see Morphine.
Dose: *Patches:* last 72 h and come in 5 strengths: 12, 25, 50, 75 and
100, which denote release of μg/h (to calculate initial dose, these are
equivalent to daily oral morphine requirement of 45, 90, 180, 270
and 360 mg, respectively).
Lozenges: initially 200 μg over 15 mins, repeating after 15 mins if
needed and adjusting dose to give max 4 dose units (available as
200, 400, 600, 800, 1200 or 1600 μg) daily.
NB: fever/external heat can ⇒ ↑absorption (∴↑fx) from patches.

FERROUS FUMARATE

As ferrous sulphate, but ↓GI upset; available in UK as Fersaday (322 mg tablet od as Px or bd as Rx), Fersamal (1–2 tablets of 210 mg tds) or Galfer (305mg capsule od/bd).

FERROUS GLUCONATE

As ferrous sulphate, but ↓GI upset. Px: 600 mg od; Rx: 1.2–1.8 g/day in 2–3 divided doses.

FERROUS SULPHATE

Oral Fe preparation.
Use: Fe-deficient ↓Hb Rx/Px.
Caution: P.
SE: dark stools (can confuse with melaena, which smells worse!), **GI upset** (esp **nausea**; consider switching to ferrous gluconate/ fumarate or take with food, but latter can ⇒ ↓absorption), Δ bowel habit (dose-dependent).
Dose: Rx: 200 mg bd/tds. Px: 200 mg od.

FINASTERIDE

Antiandrogen: 5-α-reductase inhibitor; ↓s testosterone conversion to more potent dihydrotestosterone.
Use: BPH[1] (↓s prostate size and symptoms) male-pattern baldness[2].
Caution: Ca prostate (can ⇒ ↓PSA & ∴ mask), obstructive uropathy, P (teratogenic; although not taken by women, partners of those on the drug can absorb it from handling crushed tablets and from semen, in which it is excreted ∴ *females must avoid handling tablets, and sexual partners of those on the drug must use condoms if, or likely to become, pregnant*).
SE: sexual dysfunction, testicular pain, gynaecomastia, hyper-sensitivity (inc swelling of lips/face).
Dose: 5 mg od[1] (Proscar), 1 mg od[2] (Propecia).

FLAGYL see Metronidazole; antibiotic for anaerobes

FLECAINIDE

Class Ic antiarrhythmic; local anaesthetic; ↓s conduction.

Use: VT[1] (if serious and symptomatic), SVT[2] (esp junctional re-entry tachycardias and paroxysmal AF).

CI: chronic AF (with no attempts at cardioversion), Hx of MI plus asymptomatic VEs or non-sustained VT, valvular heart disease (if haemodynamically compromised), **H**.

Caution: pacemakers, SAN dysfunction, atrial conduction dfx, AF post cardiac surgery, HB (not 1st-degree), BBB, **L/R/P/B/E**.

SE: GI upset, syncope, dyspnoea, vision/mood disturbances. Rarely **arrhythmias**.

Monitor: pre-dose plasma levels in LF or RF (keep at 0.2–1 mg/l), ECG if giving iv.

Interactions: levels ↑d by amiodarone, rito-/ampre-navir, fluoxetine and quinine. ↑s digoxin levels. Myocardial depression may occur with β-blockers/verapamil. ↑risk of arrhythmias with antipsychotics, TCAs, arthemether/lumefantrine and dolasetron.

Dose: initially 100 mg bd po, ↓ing after 3–5 days if possible (max 400 mg/day)[1]; 50 mg bd po, ↑ing if necessary to 300 mg/day[2]. Acutely, 2 mg/kg iv over 10–30 min (max 150 mg), then (if required) 1.5 mg/kg/h ivi for 1 h, then ↓ing to 100–250 μg/kg/h for up to 24 h, then give po (max cumulative dose in 1st 24 h = 600 mg).

FLEET (PHOSPHO-SODA) see Bowel preparations

Dose: 45 ml (mixed with 120 ml water, then followed by 240 ml water) taken twice: for morning procedures, at 7am and 7pm the day before; for afternoon procedures, at 7pm the day before and at 7am on the day of procedure.

FLIXOTIDE see Fluticasone (inh steroid). 50, 100, 250 or 500 μg/puff as powder. 50, 125 or 250 μg/puff as aerosol.

Dose: 100–2000 μg/day[SPC/BNF] (aerosol doses <powder doses).

FLOMAX see Tamsulosin; α₁ blocker for ↑prostate.

FLUCLOXACILLIN

Penicillin (penicillinase-resistant).
Use: penicillin-resistant (β-lactamase-producing) staphylococcal
infections, esp skin[1] (surgical wounds, iv sites, cellulitis, impetigo,
otitis externa), rarely as adjunct in pneumonia[1]. Also osteomyelitis[2],
endocarditis[3].
CI/Caution/SE/Interactions: as benzylpenicillin, plus CI if Hx
of flucloxacillin-associated jaundice/hepatic dysfunction and caution
if LF, as rarely ⇒ hepatitis or **cholestatic jaundice** (may develop
after Rx stopped).
Dose: 250–500 mg qds po/im (or up to 2 g qds iv)[1]; up to 2 g qds
iv[2]; 2 g qds (4-hrly if Wt > 85 kg) iv[3].

FLUCONAZOLE

Triazole antifungal: good po absorption and CSF penetration.
Use: fungal meningitis (esp cryptococcal), candidiasis (mucosal,
vaginal, systemic), other fungal infections (esp tinea, pittyria).
Caution: susceptibility to ↑QTc, L/R/P/B.
SE: GI upset, hypersensitivity (can ⇒ angioedema, TEN, SJS,
anaphylaxis: if develops rash, stop drug or monitor closely),
hepatotoxicity, headache. Rarely blood/metabolic (↑lipids, ↓K^+)
disorders, dizziness, seizures, alopecia.
Monitor: LFTs; stop drug if features of liver disease develop.
Interactions: ↓**P450** ∴ many; most importantly, ↑s fx of
theophyllines, ciclosporin and tacrolimus, **W+**.
Dose: 50–400 mg/day po or iv according to indication[SPC/BNF].

FLUDROCORTISONE

Mineralocorticoid (also has glucocorticoid actions).
Use: adrenocortical deficiency, esp Addison's disease[1].
CI/Caution/Interactions: See Prednisolone.
SE: H_2O/Na^+ retention, ↓K^+ (monitor U&Es). Also can ⇒
immunosuppression (and other SEs of corticosteroids; see
p. 185–6).
Dose: 50–300 µg/day po[1].

FLUMAZENIL

Benzodiazepine antagonist (competitive).

Use: benzodiazepine OD/toxicity (esp if respiratory depression).

CI: life-threatening conditions controlled by benzodiazepines (e.g. ↑ICP, status epilepticus).

Caution: mixed ODs (esp TCAs), benzodiazepine dependence (may ⇒ withdrawal fx; see p. 189), Hx of panic disorder (can ⇒ relapse), head injury, epileptics on long-term benzodiazepine Rx (may ⇒ fits), L/P/B/E.

SE: N&V, dizziness, flushing, rebound anxiety/agitation, transient ↑BP/HR.

Dose: initially 0.2 mg over 30 secs, then wait 30 secs for response. If unsuccessful give 2nd dose of 0.3 mg, then subsequent doses of 0.5 mg. *Max total dose 3 mg.*

NB: short $t_{1/2}$ (52 min); observe closely after Rx and consider further doses or ivi (at 0.1–0.5 mg/h adjusted to response).

> ☠ Flumazenil is not recommended as a diagnostic test and should not be given routinely in overdoses as risk of inducing:
>
> 1 **fits** (esp if epileptic)
> 2 **withdrawal syndrome** (if habituated to benzodiazepines)
> 3 **arrhythmias** (esp if co-ingested TCA or amphetamine-like drug). If in any doubt get senior opinion and exclude habituation to benzodiazepines and get ECG before giving unless life-threatening respiratory depression and benzodiazepine known to be cause. ☠

FLUOXETINE/PROZAC

SSRI antidepressant: long $t_{1/2}$ compared with others*.

Use: depression, other Ψ disorders (inc bulimia, OCD).

CI: active mania.

Caution: epilepsy, receiving ECT, Hx of mania or bleeding disorder (esp GI), heart disease, DM†, glaucoma (angle-closure), ↑risk of bleeding, L/R/H/P/B/E.

Class SEs: GI upset, ↓Wt, insomnia**, agitation****, headache, hypersensitivity.** Can ⇒ withdrawal fx when stopped (see p. 192) ∴ *stop slowly*; more important for SSRIs with ↓t$_{1/2}$*. Rarely extrapyramidal (see p. 192) and antimuscarinic fx (see p. 191), sexual dysfunction, convulsions, ↓Na$^+$ (inc SIADH), blood disorders, GI bleed, serotonin syndrome (see p. 192) and suicide.
Specific SEs: rarely hypoglycaemia[†], **vasculitis (rash may be 1st sign).**
Warn: can ↓performance at skilled tasks (inc driving). Don't stop suddenly (not as important as other SSRIs).
Interactions: ↓P450 ∴ many, but most importantly ↑s levels of TCAs, benzodiazepines, clozapine and haloperidol. ↑s lithium toxicity and ⇒ HTN and ↑CNS fx with selegiline (and other dopaminergics). Antagonises antiepileptics (but ↑s levels of carbamazepine and phenytoin). ☠*Never give with MAOIs.*☠ (Mild **W+**.)
Dose: 20 mg (max 60 mg) od – give mane as can ↓sleep**.

FLUTICASONE/FLIXOTIDE (various delivery devices available[BNF])
Inhaled corticosteroid for asthma: see Beclometasone.
Dose: 100–2000 μg/day inh (or 0.5–2 mg bd as nebs).
1 μg equivalent to 2 μg of beclometasone or budesonide.

FLUVASTATIN/LESCOL
HMG-CoA reductase inhibitor; 'statin' to ↓cholesterol (&TG).
Use/CI/Caution/SE/Interactions: see Simvastatin.
Dose: initially 20–40 mg od (pm or nocte). Max 80 mg/day (adjust at intervals ≥4 wks). Available in MR form (Lescol XL) at a dose of 80 mg od.

FOLIC ACID (= FOLATE)
Vitamin: building block of nucleic acids.
Use: megaloblastic ↓Hb Rx/Px if haemolysis/dialysis[1] (or GI malabsorption where ↑doses may be needed), Px against neural-tube dfx in pregnancy[2] (esp if on antiepileptics), Px of mucositis and GI upset if on methotrexate[3].
CI: malignancy (unless megaloblastic ↓Hb due to ↓folate is an important complication).

Caution: undiagnosed megaloblastic ↓Hb (i.e. ↓B$_{12}$, as found in pernicious anaemia) – *folate given without B$_{12}$ in B$_{12}$ deficiency can precipitate subacute combined degeneration of spinal cord.*
SE: malaise, bronchospasm, allergy.
Dose: 5 mg od[1] (in maintenance, ↓frequency of dose, often to weekly); 400 µg od[2] (unless mother has neural-tube defect herself or has previously had a child with a neural-tube defect, when 5 mg od needed); 5 mg once weekly[3].

FORMOTEROL (= EFORMOTEROL)/FORADIL, OXIS
Long-acting β$_2$ agonist 'LABA'; as Salmeterol plus L.
Dose: 4.5–27 µg od/bd inh (min/max doses vary with preparations[SPC/BNF]).

FOSPHENYTOIN
Antiepileptic: prodrug of phenytoin; allows safer rapid loading.
Use: epilepsy (esp status epilepticus).
CI/Caution/SE/Monitor/Warn/Interactions: as phenytoin, but ↓SEs (esp ↓arrhythmias and 'purple glove syndrome').
Dose: as phenytoin, but prescribe as 'phenytoin sodium equivalent' and note ☠**fosphenytoin 1.5 mg = phenytoin 1 mg**☠.

FRAGMIN see Dalteparin; low-molecular-weight heparin.

FRUMIL see Co-amilofruse; tablets are 5/40 (5 mg amilozide + 40 mg furosemide) unless stated as LS (2.5/20) or FORTE (10/80).

FRUSEMIDE now called furosemide

FUSIDIC ACID/FUCIDIN
Antibiotic; good bone penetration & activity against *S. aureus*.
Use: osteomyelitis, endocarditis (2° to penicillin-resistant staphylococci) – needs 2nd antibiotic to prevent resistance.
Caution: biliary disease or obstruction (⇒ ↓elimination), L/P/B.

SE: GI upset, hepatitis*. Rarely: skin/blood disorders, ARF.
Monitor: LFTs* (esp if chronic Rx, ↑doses or LF).
Dose: 500 mg tds po (↑ to 1 g tds in severe infections or
750 mg tds if using suspension); 500 mg tds iv (6–7 mg/kg tds if
Wt <50 kg).

FUROSEMIDE (previously FRUSEMIDE)

Loop diuretic: inhibits Na^+/K^+ pump in ascending loop of Henle
⇒ ↓resorption and ∴ ↑loss of $Na^+/K^+/Cl^-/H_2O$.
Use: LVF[1] (esp in acute pulmonary oedema, but also in chronic
LVF/CCF or as Px during blood transfusion), HTN, oliguria
secondary to ARF (after correcting hypovolaemia first).
CI: cirrhosis (if precomatose), **R** (if anuria).
Caution: ↓BP, ↑prostate, porphyria, L/P/B.
SE: ↓BP (inc postural), ↓K^+, ↓Na^+, ↓Ca^{2+}, ↓Mg^{2+}, ↓Cl^-
alkalosis. Also ↑**urate/gout**, GI upset, ↑glucose/impaired glucose
tolerance, ↑cholesterol/TGs (temporary). Rarely **BM suppression**
(stop drug), RF, skin reactions, pancreatitis, tinnitus/deafness (if
↑doses or RF: reversible).
Interactions: ↑s toxicity of digoxin, NSAIDs, gentamicin and
lithium. ↓s fx of antidiabetics. NSAIDs may ↓diuretic response.
Monitor: U&Es; if ↓K^+, add po K^+ supplements/K^+-sparing
diuretic or change to combination tablet (e.g. co-amilofruse).
Dose: usually 20–80 mg po/im/iv daily in divided doses. ↑doses
used in acute LVF (see p. 199) and oliguria. If HF or RF, ivi
(max 4 mg/min) can ⇒ smoother control of fluid balance[SPC/BNF]. For
blood transfusions, a rough guide is to give 20 mg with every unit if
existing LVF, and with every 2nd unit if *at risk of LVF*.

Give iv if severe oedema: if bowel oedema ⇒ ↓po absorption.

FYBOGEL

Laxative: bulking agent (ispaghula husk) for constipation (inc IBS).
CI: ↓swallow, GI obstruction, faecal impaction, colonic atony.
Dose: 1 sachet or 10 ml bd after meals with water.

Ensure good hydration, esp if elderly, GI narrowing or ↓GI motility.

L/R/H = Liver, Renal and Heart failure (full key see p. viii)

GABAPENTIN

Antiepileptic: similar structure to GABA but mechanism of action is different from drugs affecting GABA receptors.

Use: neuropathic pain[1], epilepsy[2] (adjunctive Rx of partial seizures $\pm$ 2° generalisation).

Caution: Hx of psychosis or DM, R/P/B/E.

SE: fatigue/somnolence, dizziness, cerebellar fx (esp ataxia; see p. 193), dipl-/ambly-opia, headache, rhinitis. Rarely $\downarrow$**WCC**, GI upset, arthra-/my-algia, skin reactions.

Interactions: fx $\downarrow$by antidepressants and antimalarials (csp mefloquine).

Dose: initially 300 mg od, $\uparrow$ing by 300 mg/day to max 1.8 g daily[1] or 2.4 g daily[2] in 3 divided doses (*NB: stop drug over $\geqslant$1 wk*).
Can give false-positive urinary dipstick results for proteinuria.

GELOFUSINE

Colloid plasma substitute (gelatin-based) for iv fluid resuscitation (see p. 182). 1 l contains 154 mmol Na^+ (but no K^+).

GENTAMICIN

Aminoglycoside: broad-spectrum 'cidal' antibiotic; inhibs ribosomal 30s subunit. Good Gram-negative aerobe/staphylococci cover; other organisms often need concurrent penicillin $\pm$ metronidazole.

Use: severe infections, esp sepsis, meningitis, endocarditis. Also pyelonephritis/prostatitis, biliary tract infections, pneumonia.

CI: MG*.

Caution: obesity, R/P/B/E.

SE: ototoxic, nephrotoxic (dose- and Rx length-dependent), **hypersensitivity**, rash. Rarely AAC, N&V, seizures, encephalopathy, blood disorders, myasthenia-like syndrome* (at $\uparrow$ doses; reversible), $\downarrow$$Mg^{++}$ (if prolonged Rx).

Monitor: serum levels** after 3 or 4 doses (earlier if RF).

Interactions: fx (esp toxicity) $\uparrow$ by loop diuretics (esp **furosemide**), cephalosporins, vancomycin, amphotericin, ciclosporin, tacrolimus and cytotoxics; if these drugs must be given, space doses as far from time of gentamicin dose as possible. ↑s fx of muscle relaxants and anticholinesterases. **W+**.

Dose: 3–5 mg/kg/day in 3 divided doses im/iv/ivi (od regimens possible – contact your pharmacy/microbiology dept for details); 80 mg bd iv for endocarditis Rx.

↓doses if RF (and consider if elderly or ↑↑BMI), otherwise adjust according to serum levels*: call microbiology department if unsure.

Gentamicin levels: measure peak at 1 h post-dose (ideally = 5–10 mg/l) and trough immediately predose (ideally ≤2 mg/l). Halve ideal peak levels if for endocarditis. If levels high, can ↑*spacing* of doses (as well as ↓ing *amount* of dose); as ⇒ ↑risk of ototoxicity, monitor auditory/vestibular function.
*NB: od regimens usually only require **pre-dose** level.*

GLIBENCLAMIDE

Oral antidiabetic (long-acting sulphonylurea): ↑s pancreatic insulin release – stimulates β islet cell receptors (and inhibits gluconeogenesis).

Use: type 2 DM; requires endogenous insulin to work. Not recommended for obese* (use metformin) or elderly** (use short-acting preparations, e.g. gliclazide).

CI: ketoacidosis, porphyria, **L/R** (if either severe, otherwise caution), **P/B**.

Caution: may need to replace with insulin during intercurrent illness/surgery, **E**.

SE: **hypoglycaemia** (esp in elderly**), **GI upset**, ↑**Wt***, **headache**. Rarely hypersensitivity (inc skin) reactions, blood disorders, hepatotoxicity and transient visual Δs (esp initially).

Interactions: fx ↑d by chloramphenicol, sulphonamides (inc co-trimoxazole), antifungals (esp flu-/mic-onazole), warfarin, bezafibrate and NSAIDs. Levels ↓ by rifampicin/rifabutin.

Dose: initially 5 mg mane (with food), ↑ing as necessary (max 15 mg/day).

GLICLAZIDE
Oral antidiabetic (short-acting sulphonylurea).
Use/CI/Caution/SE/Interactions: as glibenclamide, but shorter action* and hepatic metabolism** mean ↓d risk of hypoglycaemia (esp in elderly* and RF**).
Dose: initially 40–80 mg mane (with food), ↑ing as necessary (max 320 mg/day). MR tablets available (Diamicron MR) of which 30 mg has equivalent effect as 80 mg of normal release (dose initially is 30 mg od, ↑ing if necessary to max 120 mg od).

GLIMEPIRIDE
Oral antidiabetic (short-acting sulphonylurea).
Use/CI/Caution/SE/Interactions: as gliclazide, plus manufacturer recommends monitoring of FBC & LFTs.
Dose: initially 1 mg mane (with food), ↑ing as necessary (max 6 mg/day).

GLIPIZIDE
Oral antidiabetic (short-acting sulphonylurea).
Use/CI/Caution/SE/Interactions: as gliclazide.
Dose: initially 2.5–5.0 mg mane (with food), ↑ing as necessary (max single dose 15 mg; max daily dose 20 mg).

GLIQUIDONE
Oral antidiabetic (short-acting sulphonylurea).
Use/CI/Caution/SE/Interactions: as gliclazide.
Dose: initially 15 mg mane (with food), ↑ing as necessary (max single dose 60 mg, max daily dose 180 mg).

GLUCAGON
Polypeptide hormone: ↑s hepatic glycogen conversion to glucose.
Use: hypoglycaemia: if acute and severe, esp if no iv access or if 2° to xs insulin (see p. 206).
CI: phaeo.
Caution: glucagonomas/insulinomas. Will not work if hypo-glycaemia is chronic (inc starvation) or 2° to adrenal insufficiency.

SE: N&V&D, ↓BP, ↓K$^+$, hypersensitivity, **W+**.
Dose: 1 mg (= 1 unit) **im** (or sc/iv).
Often stocked in cardiac arrest ('crash') trolleys.

GLYCEROL (= GLYCERIN) SUPPOSITORIES

Rectal irritant bowel stimulant.
Use: constipation: 1st-line suppository if oral methods such as lactulose and senna fail.
Dose: 1–2 pr prn.

GLYCERYL TRINITRATE see GTN

GRANISETRON

Antiemetic: 5HT$_3$ antagonist.
Use: N&V; see Ondansetron.
Caution: GI obstruction (inc subacute), P/B.
SE: constipation (or diarrhoea), **headache**, sedation, fatigue, dizziness. Rarely seizures, chest pain, ↓BP, Δ LFTs, rash, hypersensitivity.
Dose: 1 mg bd or 2 mg od po/iv/ivi for non-specialist use. 2–3 mg loading doses often given before chemotherapy$^{SPC/BNF}$ (max 9 mg/24 h).

GTN (= GLYCERYL TRINITRATE)

Nitrate: ⇒ coronary artery + systemic vein dilation ⇒ ↑O$_2$ supply to myocardium and ↓preload, ∴ ↓O$_2$ demand of myocardium.
Use: Angina, LVF.
CI: ↓BP, ↓↓Hb, aortic/mitral stenosis, constrictive pericarditis, tamponade, HOCM, glaucoma (closed-angle), hypovolaemia, ↑ICP.
Caution: recent MI, ↓T$_4$, hypothermia, head trauma, cerebral haemorrhage, malnutrition, L/R (if either severe).
SE: ↓BP (inc postural), **headache**, dizziness, flushing, ↑HR.
Interactions: ☠sildenafil, tadalafil and vardenafil (are CI as ⇒ ↓↓BP). ☠ ↓s fx of heparins (if given iv).

Dose: 2 sprays or tablets sl prn (also available as transdermal SR patches[SPC/BNF]). For acute MI/LVF: 10–200 µg/min ivi, titrating to clinical response and BP (see pp. 196–7).

HALOPERIDOL

Butyrophenone ('typical') antipsychotic: dopamine antagonist ($D_{2\&3} > D_{1\&4}$). Also blocks serotonin ($5HT_{2A}$), histamine (H_1), adrenergic ($\alpha_{1>2}$) and muscarinic receptors, causing many SEs.

Use: acute sedation[1] (e.g. agitation, behavioural disturbance – esp in elderly and Ψ disorders), schizophrenia[2], N&V[3].

CI/Caution/SE: as chlorpromazine, but ⇒ ↑incidence of **extrapyramidal fx**, although ⇒ ↓sedation, ↓skin reactions, ↓antimuscarinic fx, ↓BP fx, but can ⇒ hypoglycaemia and SIADH.

Interactions: **metabolised by P450** ∴ many, but most importantly: levels ↑by fluoxetine, venlafaxine, quinidine, buspirone and ritonavir. Levels ↓by carbamazepine, phenytoin, rifampicin. ↑risk of arrhythmias with amiodarone and ↓s fx of anticonvulsants.

Dose: 1.5–5.0 mg bd/tds po (max 30 mg/day)[1,2]; 2–10 mg im/iv 4–8-hourly (max 18 mg/day)[1,2]; 0.5–2.0 mg tds im/iv[3]. Also uscd im as a 4-wkly 'depot'[2] if concerns over compliance.

Start at bottom of dose range if naive to antipsychotics, esp if elderly. See pp. 187–8 for advice on acute sedation.

HARTMANN'S SOLUTION

Compound sodium lactate iv fluid; used mostly in surgery and trauma. 1 l contains **5 mmol K^+**, 2 mmol Ca^{2+}, 29 mmol HCO_3^-, 131 mmol Na^+, 111 mmol Cl^-.

HELICLEAR

Triple-therapy combination preparation of PPI and two antibiotics.

Use: *H. pylori* eradication.

CI/Caution/SE/Interactions: as per individual drugs.

Dose: lansoprazole 30 mg bd + amoxicillin 1 g bd + clarithromycin 500 mg bd for 7–14 days.

HEPARIN, standard/unfractionated (NB: ≠ LMWHs).

iv (and rarely sc) anticoagulant: potentiates protease inhibitor antithrombin III, which inactivates thrombin. Also inhibits factors IXa/Xa/XIa/XIIa.

Use: anticoagulation if needs to be immediate or quickly reversible (only as inpatient); DVT/PE Rx/Px (inc preoperative), MI/unstable angina Rx/Px, extracorporeal circuits (esp haemodialysis, cardiopulmonary bypass).

CI: haemorrhagic disorders (inc haemophilia), ↓Pt (inc Hx of HIT*), severe HTN, PU, acute bacterial endocarditis, recent cerebral haemorrhage or major surgery/trauma to eye/brain/spinal cord, epidural/spinal anaesthesia (but can give Px doses), **L** (if severe, esp if oesophageal varices).

Caution: ↑K^{+}**, R/P/E.

SE: haemorrhage, ↓Pt* (HIT*), **hypersensitivity** (inc anaphylaxis, urticaria, angioedema), ↑K^{+}** (inhibits aldosterone: ↑risk if DM, CRF, acidosis or on K^{+}-sparing drugs), osteoporosis (if prolonged Rx).

Monitor: FBC* if >5 days Rx, U&E** if > 7 days Rx.

Interactions: fx may ↓by GTN ivi. NSAIDs ⇒ ↑bleeding risk.

Dose: see pp. 175–7 (inc dose-adjustment advice).

☠HIT* **H**eparin **I**nduced **T**hrombocytopenia: immune mediated ∴ delayed onset – ↑risk if Rx for >5 days (see p. 175).☠

HUMALOG see Insulin lispro; short-acting recombinant insulin. Also available as biphasic preparations (Mix 25, Mix 50) are combined with longer-acting isophane suspension.

HUMULIN recombinant insulin available in various forms:

1   HUMULIN S soluble, short-acting for iv/acute use (DKA/sliding scales).
2   HUMULIN I isophane (combined with protamine), long-acting.

3 HUMULIN M 'biphasic' preparations, combination of short-acting (S) and long-acting (I) forms to give smoother control throughout the day. Numbers denote 1/10 of the percentage of soluble insulin (i.e. M2 = 20%, M3 = 30%, M5 = 50% soluble insulin).

HYDRALAZINE

Antihypertensive: vasodilates smooth muscle (arteries >veins).
Use: HTN[1] (inc severe[2], esp if RF or pregnancy), HF[3].
CI: severe ↑HR, myocardial insufficiency (2° mechanical obstruction, e.g. aortic/mitral stenosis or constrictive pericarditis T[4]), SLE*, porphyria, **H** (if "high output", e.g. ↑T[4]).
Caution: IHD, cerebrovascular disease, L/R/P/B.
SE: (all SEs ↓if dose <100 mg/day) ↑**HR, GI upset, headache, lupus-like syndrome*** (watch for unexplained ↓Wt, arthritis, ill health – measure ANA* and dipstick urine for protein if on high doses/clinical suspicion). Also fluid retention (↓d if used with diuretics), palpitations, dizziness, flushing, ↓BP (even at low doses), blood disorders, arthr-/my-algia, rash and can worsen IHD.
Dose: 25–50 mg bd po[1]; 5–10 mg iv[2] (can be repeated after 20–30 min) or 50–300 µg/min ivi[2]; 25–75 mg tds/qds po[3].

HYDROCORTISONE BUTYRATE CREAM (0.1%)

Potent-strength topical corticosteroid. *NB: much stronger than 'standard' (i.e. non-butyrate) hydrocortisone cream; see below!*

HYDROCORTISONE CREAM (1%)

Mild-strength topical corticosteroid (rarely used as weaker 0.5%, 0.25% and 0.1% preparations).

HYDROCORTISONE iv/po

Glucocorticoid (with significant mineralocorticoid activity).
Use: acute hypersensitivity (esp anaphylaxis, angioedema), Addisonian crisis, asthma, COPD, ↓T[4] (and ↑T[4]), IBD. Also used po in chronic adrenocortical deficiency.
CI/Caution/SE/Interactions: see pp. 185–7.

Dose: *acutely:* 100–300 mg im or slowly iv up to qds if required. Exact dose recommendations vary: consult local protocol if unsure (see Medical emergencies section of this book for rational starting dose for some specific indications). *Chronic replacement:* usually 20–30 mg po daily in divided doses (usually 2/3 in morning and 1/3 nocte), often together with fludrocortisone.

HYDROXOCOBALAMIN

Vitamin B_{12} replacement.
Use: pernicious anaemia (also macrocytic anaemias with neurological involvement, tobacco amblyopia, Leber's optic atrophy).
SE: skin reactions, GI upset, 'flu-like symptoms, $\downarrow K^+$ (initially), rarely anaphylaxis.
Interactions: fx $\downarrow$by OCP and chloramphenicol.
Dose: 1 mg im injection: frequently at first for Rx (3–7/wk: exact number depends on indication[SPC/BNF]) until no further improvement, then $\downarrow$frequency (to once every 1–3 months) for maintenance.

HYDROXYCARBAMIDE (= HYDROXYUREA)

Oral agent for CML. 2nd-line Rx for polycythaemia, severe psoriasis.
SE: GI upset, blood disorders (esp **myelosuppression**), skin reactions.
CI/Caution: see SPC.
Dose: 20–30 mg/kg daily (or 80 mg/kg every 3rd day). Specialist use only.

HYOSCINE BUTYLBROMIDE/BUSCOPAN

Antimuscarinic: $\downarrow$s GI motility. Doesn't cross BBB (unlike hyoscine *hydrobromide*) $\therefore$ less sedative.
Use: GI (or GU) smooth-muscle spasm; esp biliary colic, diverticulitis and IBS. Rarely used for dysmenorrhoea.
CI/Caution/SE: As atropine, plus CI in megacolon.
Interactions: $\downarrow$fx of metoclopramide and vice versa. $\uparrow$s tachycardic fx of β-agonists.
Dose: 20 mg qds po (for IBS, start at 10 mg tds) or 20 mg im/iv (repeating once after 30 min, if necessary; max 100 mg/day).
Don't confuse with hyoscine *hydrobromide*: different fx and doses!

HYOSCINE HYDROBROMIDE (= SCOPOLAMINE)

Antimuscarinic: predominant fx on CNS ($\downarrow$s vestibular activity[1]). Also $\downarrow$s respiratory/oral secretions[2,3].

Use: motion sickness[1], terminal care/chronic $\downarrow$swallow[2] (e.g. CVA), hypersalivation 2° to antipsychotics[3] (unlicensed use).

CI: glaucoma (closed-angle).

Caution: GI obstruction, $\uparrow$prostate/urinary retention, cardiovascular disease, porphyria, Down's, MG, L/R/P/B/E.

SE: antimuscarinic fx (see p. 191), generally sedative (although rarely $\Rightarrow$ paradoxical agitation when given as sc infusion).

Warn: driving may be impaired, $\uparrow$s fx of alcohol.

Interactions: $\downarrow$s fx of sublingual nitrates (e.g. GTN).

Dose: 300 µg 6-hrly po (max 3 doses/24 h)[1] (or as transdermal patches; release 1 mg over 72 h); 0.6–2.4 mg/24 h as sc infusion[2] (see p. 157 for use in palliative care); 300 µg bd po[3] (can $\uparrow$ to qds).

Don't confuse with hyoscine *butylbromide*: different fx and doses!

HYPROMELLOSE 0.3% EYE DROPS

Artificial tears for Sjogren's/other causes of dry eyes.

Dose: 1–2 drops prn (often given with the mucolytic acetylcysteine for filamentary keratitis). Also available in 0.5% or 1% solutions[SPC/BNF].

IBUGEL/IBULEVE ibuprofen topical gel/spray respectively for musculoskeletal pain.

IBUPROFEN

NSAID (propionic acid derivative): unselective COX inhibitor; anti-inflammatory, antipyrexial[†] and analgesic properties.

Use: mild/moderate pain[1] (headache, gynaecological/musculoskeletal pain; not 1st choice for gout/rheumatoid arthritis), fever[2], mild local inflammation[3].

CI: Hx of hypersensitivity to any NSAID (inc asthma, angioedema, urticaria or rhinitis reactions). Hx of, or active, peptic ulcer*.

Caution: Hx of asthma, GI disease, $\uparrow$BP or allergic disorders, coagulopathy. *Can mask signs of infection*[†]. L/R/H/P/B/E.

SE: (*generally milder than with other NSAIDs*) **GI upset/ ulceration*/bleeding**. Also headache, nervousness, dizziness, fluid retention/oedema, ARF, hypersensitivity reactions (esp bronchospasm and skin reactions, inc SJS/TEN). Rarely, blood disorders, ↑BP.
Interactions: ↓s fx of antihypertensives, ↑s (toxic) fx of methotrexate, AZT, tacrolimus, digoxin, quinolones and lithium. ↑risk of RF with ACE-i, ARB and ciclosporin (mild **W+**).
Dose: 200–400 mg tds po[1&2] (↑dose needed for rheumatoid arthritis: up to 800 mg tds); topically as gel[3].

IMODIUM see Loperamide; antimotility agent for diarrhoea.

INDAPAMIDE

Thiazide derivative diuretic; see Bendroflumethiazide.
Use: HTN.
CI: Hx of sulphonamide derivative allergy, **L** (if severe).
Caution: ↑PTH (stop if ↑Ca^{2+}), ↑aldosterone, gout, **R/P/B/E**.
SE: as bendroflumethiazide, but reportedly fewer metabolic disturbances (esp less hyperglycaemia).
Monitor: U&Es, urate.
Interactions: ↑s lithium levels and toxicity of digoxin (if ⟹ ↓K$^+$).
Dose: 2.5 mg od mane (or 1.5 mg od of SR preparation).

INDOMETACIN

High-strength NSAID: unselective COX inhibitor.
Use: musculoskeletal pain[1]; esp gout, ankylosing spondylitis, rheumatoid arthritis, dysmennorhoea (use limited by SEs*). Also used in specialist setting for PDA closure.
CI/Caution/SE/Interactions: as ibuprofen, but ↑incidence of SEs, esp GI bleeding, headaches, dizziness, Ψ disturbances (all of which are dose-dependent). Also caution in epilepsy and parkinsonism.
Dose: 25–50 mg up to qds po or 100 mg up to bd pr (max total daily dose 200 mg)[1]. Use high end of this dose range for gout, and ↓dose once pain under control. SR preparations available[SPC/BNF] (75–200 mg/day in 1–2 divided doses).

▼INFLIXIMAB/REMICADE

Monoclonal Ab against TNF-α (inflammatory cytokine).

Use: Crohn's, RA, psoriasis (for skin or arthritis) or ankylosing spondylitis resistant to steroids/immunosuppression[NICE].

CI: TB or other severe infections, **H** (unless mild when only caution), **P/B**.

Caution: infections, demyelinating CNS disorders, **L/R**.

SE: severe infections, TB (inc extrapulmonary), **CCF** (exac of), **CNS demyelination**. Also GI upset, 'flu-like symptoms, cough, fatigue, headache. ↑incidence of hypersensitivity (esp transfusion) reactions.

Dose: specialist use only.

IODINE and IODIDE see Lugol's solution; used for ↑↑T_4.

INSULATARD long-acting (isophane) insulin, either recombinant human or porcine.

INSULIN see pp. 166–71 for different types and prescribing advice.

INTEGRILIN see Eptifibatide; anti Pt agent for IIID.

IPOCOL see Mesalazine; 'new' aminosalicylate for UC, with ↓SEs.

IPRATROPIUM

Inh muscarinic antagonist; bronchodilator and ↓s bronchial secretions.

Use: chronic[1] and acute[2] bronchospasm (COPD >asthma). Rarely used topically for rhinitis.

SE: antimuscarinic fx (see p. 191), usually minimal.

Caution: glaucoma (angle closure only; protect patient's eyes from drug, esp if giving nebs: use tight-fitting mask), bladder outflow obstruction (e.g. ↑prostate), **P/B**.

Dose: 20–40 µg tds/qds inh[1] (max 80 µg qds); 250–500 µg qds neb[2] (↑ing up to 4-hourly if severe).

IRBESARTAN/APROVEL

Angiotensin II antagonist.

Use: HTN, type 2 DM nephropathy.

CI: P/B.

Caution/SE/Interactions: see Losartan.
Dose: initially 150 mg od, ↑ing to 300 mg od if required (halve initial dose if age >75 years or on haemodialysis).

IRON TABLETS see Ferrous sulphate/fumarate/gluconate

ISDN see Isosorbide dinitrate

ISMN see Isosorbide mononitrate

ISMO see Isosorbide mononitrate

ISONIAZID

Antituberculous antibiotic; 'static'.
Use: TB (see p. 143).
CI: drug-induced liver disease.
Caution: Hx of psychosis/epilepsy/porphyria or if ↑d risk of neuropathy[†] (e.g. DM, alcohol abuse, CRF, malnutrition, HIV: give pyridoxine 10–20 mg od as Px), porphyria, L/R/P/B.
SE: optic neuritis, peripheral neuropathy[†], hepatitis*, rash, gynaecomastia, GI upset. Rarely lupus, blood disorders (inc rarely agranulocytosis[**]), hypersensitivity, convulsions, psychosis.
Warn: patient of symptoms of liver disease and to seek medical help if they occur.
Monitor: LFTs*, FBC[**].
Interactions: ↓P450 ∴ many, but most importantly ↑s levels of carbamazepine, phenytoin, ethosuximide and benzodiazepines **W+**.
Dose: by weight[SPC/BNF] or as combination preparation (see p. 143). Take on empty stomach (⩾30 min before or ⩾2 h after meal).
Acetylator-dependent metabolism: if slow acetylator ⇒ ↑risk of SEs.

ISOSORBIDE DINITRATE (ISDN)

Nitrate; as GTN, but available po as well as sl.
Use/CI/Caution/SE/Interactions: as GTN, but ⇒ ↓headache.
Dose: 1.25–2.5 mg (1–2 sprays) sl prn; 10–80 mg tds po, titrating up slowly (bd MR preparations available[SPC/BNF]); 2–20 mg/h ivi (write up similarly to GTN on pp. 196–7, i.e. 50 mg made up to 50 ml at 0–10 ml/h).

Sublingual preparations of ISDN degrade less over time than those of GTN and ∴ better for those who need nitrates infrequently (less drug ends up being thrown away!)

ISOSORBIDE MONONITRATE (ISMN)
Nitrate; as GTN, but po rather than sl delivery.
Use/CI/Caution/SE/Interactions: as GTN, but ⇒ ↓headache.
Dose: 10–40 mg bd/tds po (od MR preparations available^SPC/BNF).

ISTIN see Amlodipine; Ca^{2+} channel blocker for HTN/IHD.

ITRACONAZOLE/SPORANOX
Triazole antifungal: needs acidic pH for good po absorption*.
Use: fungal infections (candida, tinea, cryptococcus, aspergillosis, histoplasmosis, onychomycosis, pityriasis versicolor).
Caution: risk of HF: Hx of cardiac disease or if on negative inotropic drugs (risk ↑s with dose, length of Rx and age), L/R/P/B.
SE: HF, hepatotoxicity, GI upset, headache**, dizziness, peripheral neuropathy (if occurs, stop drug), cholestasis, menstrual Δs, skin reactions (inc angioedema, SJS). With prolonged Rx can ⇒ ↓K^+, oedema, hair loss.
Monitor: LFTs** if Rx >1 month or Hx of (or develop clinical features of) liver disease: stop drug if become abnormal.
Interactions: ↓P450 ∴ many; most importantly ↑s risk of **myopathy with statins** (avoid together) and ↑s risk of **HF with negative inotropes** (esp Ca^{2+} blockers). ↑s fx of ☠ **midazolam, quinidine, pimozide** ☠, ciclosporin, digoxin, indinavir and siro-/ tacro-limus. fx ↓d by rifampicin, phenytoin and **antacids***, W+.
Dose: dependent on indication^SPC/BNF. *Take with food.*

KAY-CEE-L
KCl syrup (1 mmol/ml).
Use: ↓K^+.
CI/Caution/SE: as Sando-K.

Dose: according to serum K$^+$: average 25–50 ml/day if diet normal (↓ if renal impairment).

KETOCONAZOLE/NIZORAL

Imidazole antifungal: good po absorption.

Use: fungal infection Rx (if systemic, severe or resistant to topical Rx) and Px if immunosuppression.

CI: L/P/B.

Caution: porphyria.

SE: ☠hepatitis* ☠, GI upset, **skin reactions** (rash, urticaria, pruritus, photosensitivity, rarely angioedema), **gynaecomastia**, blood disorders, paraesthesia, dizziness, photophobia.

Monitor: LFTs*, esp if Rx >14 days.

Interactions: ↓P450 ∴ many; most importantly, ↑s risk of **myopathy with statins** (avoid together). ↑s fx of ☠**midazolam, quinidine, pimozide**☠, vardenafil, eplerenone, cilostazol, reboxetine, aripiprazole, sertindole, felodipine, ergot alkaloids, antidiabetics, buprenorphine, artemether/lumefantrine, indi-/rito-navir and ciclosporin (and possibly theophyllines). ↓s fx of rifampicin (rifampicin can also ↓ fx of ketoconazole, as can phenytoin), **W+**.

Dose: 200 mg od po *with food* (400 mg od in severe/resistant cases).

KLEAN-PREP see Bowel preparations

Dose: up to 2 powder sachets the evening before and repeated on the morning of GI surgery or Ix.

KLOREF

Effervescent oral KCl (6.7 mmol K$^+$/tablet).

Use: ↓K$^+$.

CI/Caution/SE: as Sando-K.

Dose: according to serum K$^+$: average 4–8 tablets/day if diet normal (↓ if renal impairment).

LABETALOL

β-blocker with arteriolar vasodilatory properties ∴ also ⇒ ↓TPR.

Use: severe HTN (inc during pregnancy[1] or post-MI[2] or with angina).

CI/Caution/SE/Interactions: as propranolol, plus can $\Rightarrow$ ☠ **severe/postural $\downarrow$BP** ☠ and hepatotoxicity* (L).
Monitor: LFTs (if deteriorate stop drug).
Dose: initially 100 mg bd po (halve dose in elderly), $\uparrow$ing every fortnight if necessary to max of 600 mg qds po; if essential to $\downarrow$BP rapidly give 50 mg iv over $\geq$ 1 min repeating after 5 min if necessary (or can give 2 mg/min ivi), up to max total dose 200 mg; 20 mg/h ivi[1], doubling every 30 min to max of 160 mg/h; 15 mg/h ivi[2], $\uparrow$ing slowly to max of 120 mg/h.

LACRI-LUBE

Artificial tears for dry eyes.
SE: blurred vision.
Dose: 1–2 drops prn (best used nocte).

LACTULOSE

Osmotic laxative[1]: semisynthetic disaccharide bulking agent. Also $\downarrow$s growth of NH_4-producing bacteria[2].
Use: constipation[1], hepatic encephalopathy[2].
CI: GI obstruction, galactosaemia.
Caution: lactose intolerance.
SE: flatulence, distension, abdominal pains.
Dose: 15 ml od/bd[1] ($\uparrow$dose according to response; NB: *can take 2 days to work*); 30–50 ml tds[2].

LAMOTRIGINE/LAMICTAL

Antiepileptic: $\downarrow$s release of excitatory amino acids (esp glutamate) via action on voltage-sensitive Na^+ channels
Use: epilepsy (esp partial and 1° or 2° generalised tonic–clonic).
Caution: avoid abrupt withdrawal† (rebound seizure risk; taper off over $\geq$2 wks unless stopping due to serious skin reaction*), L/R/P/B/E.
SE: cerebellar symptoms (see p. 193), **skin reactions*** (often severe, e.g. SJS, TEN, lupus, esp in children or if also on valproate), **blood disorders**** ($\downarrow$Hb, $\downarrow$WCC, $\downarrow$Pt), N&V. Rarely, $\downarrow$memory, sedation, Ψ disorders, sleep Δ, acne, pretibial ulcers, alopecia, worsening of seizures, poly-/an-uria, **hepatotoxicity**.
Monitor: U&Es, FBC, LFTs, clotting.

Warn: report rash* plus any 'flu-like symptoms, signs of infection/↓Hb or bruising**. Don't stop tablets suddenly†.
Interactions: fx are ↓d by OCP, phenytoin, carbamazepine, mefloquine, TCAs and SSRIs. fx ↑d by valproate.
Dose: 25–700 mg daily[SPC/BNF]; ↑dose slowly to ↓risk of skin reactions* (also need to restart at low dose).

LANSOPRAZOLE/ZOTON
PPI. As omeprazole, but ↓ interactions.
Dose: 15–30 mg od po (↓ to 15 mg od for maintenance).

LARIAM see Mefloquine; antimalarial (Px and Rx).

LATANOPROST/XALATAN
Topical PG analogue: ↑s uveoscleral outflow.
Use: ↑IOP in glaucoma (open-angle) and *ocular* HTN.
CI: use of all contact lenses.
Caution: asthma (if severe), aphakia, pseudophakia, P/B.
SE: blurred vision, local reactions, ↑s brown pigmentation of iris (warn patient of this). Rarely cystoid macular oedema, uveitis, angina.
Dose: 1 drop od (nocte) of 50-µg/ml solution.

LASIX see Furosemide; loop diuretic.

▼LEFLUNOMIDE/ARAVA
DMARD; inhibits pyrimidine synthesis (also anti-inflammatory fx).
Use: moderate/severe active rheumatoid arthritis if standard DMARDs (e.g. methotrexate or sulfasalazine) CI or not tolerated.
CI: severe immunodeficiency, BM suppression, severe hypoproteinaemia, serious infection, **L/R/P/B**.
Caution: blood disorders, recent hepato-/myelo-toxic drugs, TB (inc Hx of).
SE: BM toxicity, ↑risk of **infection/malignancy**, hepatotoxicity, HTN.
Warn: teratogenic: must exclude pregnancy before starting Rx and use contraception during Rx (and until drug no longer active*).
Monitor: LFTs, FBC, BP.

L/R/H = Liver, Renal and Heart failure (full key see p. viii)

Dose: specialist use only.

Long $t_{1/2}$*: needs prolonged washout period or active measures (e.g. cholestyramine 8 g tds or activated charcoal 50 g qds) to ↑elimination if wishing to conceive.

LEVOBUNOLOL

β-blocker eye drops: similar to timolol ⇒ ↓aqueous humour production. *Significant systemic absorption can occur.*
Use: chronic simple (wide/open angle) glaucoma.
CI/Caution/Interactions: as propranolol; interactions less likely.
SE: local reactions. Rarely anterior uveitis and anaphylaxis. Can ⇒ systemic fx, esp bronchoconstriction and cardiac fx; see Propranolol.
Dose: 1 drop of 0.5% solution od/bd.

LEVODOPA (= L-DOPA)

Precursor of dopamine: needs concomitant peripheral dopa decarboxylase inhibitor such as benserazide (see Co-beneldopa) or carbidopa (see Co-careldopa) to limit SEs.
Use: parkinsonism.
CI: glaucoma (closed-angle), taking MAOIs*, melanoma[†], **P/B**.
Caution: pulmonary/cardiovascular/Ψ disease, DM, glaucoma (open angle), osteomalacia, Hx of PU or convulsions, L/R.
SE: dyskinesias, abdominal upset, postural ↓BP, drowsiness, aggression, Ψ disorders (confusion, depression, suicide, hallucinations, psychosis, hypomania), seizures, dizziness, headache, flushing, sweating, peripheral neuropathy, taste Δs, rash/pruritus, can reactivate melanoma[†], Δ LFTs, GI bleeding, blood disorders, dark body fluids (inc sweat).
Warn: can ⇒ daytime sleepiness (inc sudden-onset sleep) and ↓ability to drive/operate machinery.
Interactions: fx ↓d by neuroleptics, SEs ↑d by bupropion, **risk of ↑BP crisis with MAOIs***, risk of arrhythmias with halothane.
Dose: 125–500 mg daily, *after food*, ↑ing according to response.

Abrupt withdrawal can ⇒ neuroleptic malignant-like syndrome.

LEVOMEPROMAZINE (= METHOTRIMEPRAZINE)

Phenothiazine antipsychotic; as chlorpromazine, but used in palliative care (see p. 157) as has good antiemetic[1] and sedative[2] fx, but little respiratory depression.
Use: refractory N&V[1] or restlessness/distress[2] in the terminally ill.
CI/Caution/SE/Interactions: as chlorpromazine, but ↑risk of postural ↓**BP** (esp in elderly: don't give if age >50 years and ambulant).
Dose: 12.5–25 mg im/iv tds/qds, or 25–200 mg/24 h sc infusion.
NB: for N&V low doses may be effective and ⇒ ↓sedation.

LEVOTHYROXINE see Thyroxine

LIBRIUM see Chlordiazepoxide; long-acting benzodiazepine.

LIDOCAINE (previously LIGNOCAINE)

Class Ib antiarrhythmic (↓s conduction in Purkinje and ventricular muscle fibres), local anaesthetic (blocks axonal Na$^+$ channels).
Use: ventricular arrhythmias (esp post-MI), local anaesthesia.
CI: myocardial depression (if severe), SAN disorders, atrio-ventricular block (all grades), porphyria.
Caution: epilepsy, severe hypoxia/hypovolaemia/↓HR, **L/H/P/B/E**.
SE: dizziness, drowsiness, confusion, tinnitus, blurred vision, paraesthesia, GI upset, arrhythmias, ↓BP, ↓HR. Rarely respiratory depression, seizures, hypersensitivity.
Monitor: ECG during iv administration.
Interactions: ↑risk of arrhythmias with antipsychotics, dolasetron and quinu-/dalfo-pristin. ↑myocardial depression with other antiarrhythmics and β-blockers. Levels ↑by propranolol, ampre-/ataza-/lopi-navir and cimetidine. Prolongs action of suxamethonium.
Dose (for *arrhythmias*): 50–100 mg iv at rate of 25–30 mg/min followed immediately by ivi at 4 mg/min for 30 min then 2 mg/min for 2 h and 1 mg/min thereafter (↓dose further if drug needed for >24 h). NB: short t$_{1/2}$ ∴ if 15 min delay in setting up ivi, can give max 2 further doses of 50–100 mg iv ≥ 10 min apart. In

emergencies, can often be found stocked in crash trolleys as Minijet syringes of 1% (10 mg/ml) or 2% (20 mg/ml) solutions.

💀 Local anaesthetic preparations must never be injected into veins or inflamed tissue, as can ⇒ systemic fx (esp arrhythmias). 💀

LIGNOCAINE see Lidocaine

LIOTHYRONINE (= L-TRI-IODOTHYRONINE) SODIUM

Synthetic T_3: quicker and more potent action than thyroxine (T_4).
Use: acute hypothyroidism (e.g. myxoedema coma*: see p. 207).
CI/Caution/SE/Interactions: see Thyroxine.
Dose: 5–20 μg iv slowly. Repeat every 4–12 h as necessary; seek expert help. Also available po, but thyroxine (T_4) often preferred.
Concurrent hydrocortisone iv is often also needed*; see p. 207.

LISINOPRIL

ACE-i; see Captopril.
Use: HTN[1], HF[2], Px of IHD post-MI[3], DM nephropathy[4].
CI/Caution/SE/Interactions: as Captopril.
Dose: initially 10 mg od[1] (2.5–5.0 mg if RF or used with diuretic) ↑ing if necessary to max 80 mg/day; initially 2.5 mg od[2,4] adjusted to response to usual maintenance of 5–20 mg/day. Doses post-MI depend on BP[SPC/BNF].

LITHIUM

Mood stabiliser: mechanism not fully understood; blocks neuronal Ca^{2+} channels and changes GABA pathways.
Use: mania Rx/Px, bipolar disorder Px. Rarely for recurrent depression Px and aggressive/self-mutilating behaviour Rx.
CI: ↓T_4 (if untreated), Addison's, SSS, cardiovascular disease, **P** (⇒ Ebstein's anomaly: esp in 1st trimester), **R/H/B**.
(NB: manufacturers don't agree on definitive list and all CI are **relative** – decisions should be made in clinical context and expert help sought if unsure.)
Caution: thyroid disease, MG, **E**.

SE: thirst, polyuria, GI upset ($\uparrow$Wt, N&V&D), *fine* tremor* (NB: in toxicity $\Rightarrow$ *coarse* tremor), tardive dyskinesia, muscular weakness, acne, psoriasis exacerbation, $\uparrow$WCC, $\uparrow$Pt. Rarer but serious: $\downarrow$ (or $\uparrow$) T$_4$ $\pm$ goitre (esp in females); renal impairment (diabetes insipidus, interstitial nephritis), arrhythmias.

Monitor: serum levels *12 h post-dose:* keep at 0.6–1.0 mmol/l (>1.5 mmol/l may $\Rightarrow$ toxicity, esp if elderly), U&Es, TFTs.

Warn: report symptoms of $\downarrow$T$_4$, avoid dehydration.

Interactions: toxicity ($\pm$ levels) $\uparrow$d by **NSAIDs, diuretics**** (esp thiazides), SSRIs, ACE-i, ARBs, amiodarone, methyldopa, carbamazepine and haloperidol. Theophyllines, caffeine and antacids may $\downarrow$ lithium levels.

Dose: see SPC/BNF: 2 *types* (salts) available with different doses ('carbonate' 200 mg = 'citrate' 509 mg) and bioavailabilities of particular *brands* vary $\therefore$ *must specify salt and brand required.* Consider stopping 24 h before major surgery; restart once e'lytes return to normal. Discuss with anaesthetist $\pm$ psychiatrist.

> **Lithium toxicity**
> *Features:* D&V, coarse tremor*, cerebellar signs (see p. 193), renal impairment/oliguria, $\downarrow$BP, $\uparrow$reflexes, convulsions, drowsiness $\Rightarrow$ coma. *Rx:* stop drug, control seizures, correct electrolytes (normally need saline ivi; high risk if $\downarrow$Na$^+$: avoid low-salt diets and diuretics**). Consider haemodialysis if RF.

LOCOID see Hydrocortisone butyrate 0.1% (potent steroid) cream

LOPERAMIDE/IMODIUM

Antimotility agent: synthetic opioid analogue; binds to receptors in GI muscle $\Rightarrow$ $\downarrow$peristalsis, $\uparrow$transit time, $\uparrow$H$_2$O/electrolyte resorption, $\downarrow$gut secretions, $\uparrow$sphincter tone. Extensive 1st-pass metabolism $\Rightarrow$ minimal systemic opioid fx.

Use: diarrhoea.

CI: constipation, ileus, megacolon, bacterial enterocolitis 2° to invasive organisms (e.g. salmonella, shigella, campylobacter), abdominal distension, active UC/AAC.

L/R/H = Liver, Renal and Heart failure (full key see p. viii)

Caution: in young (can ⇒ fluid + electrolyte depletion), **L/P**.
SE: constipation, abdominal cramps, bloating, dizziness, drowsiness, fatigue. Rarely hypersensitivity (esp skin reactions), paralytic ileus.
Dose: initially 4 mg, then 2 mg after each loose stool (max 16 mg/day for 5 days). *NB: can mask serious conditions.*

LORATADINE
Non-sedating antihistamine: see Cetirizine.
Dose: 10 mg od. Non-proprietary or as Clarityn.

LORAZEPAM
Benzodiazepine, short-acting (see p. 190).
Use: sedation[1] (esp acute behavioural disturbance/Ψ disorders, e.g. acute psychosis), status epilepticus[2].
CI/Caution/SE/Interactions: see Diazepam.
Dose: 0.5–2 mg po/im/iv prn (bottom of this range if elderly/respiratory disease/naive to benzodiazepines; top of range if young/recent exposure to benzodiazepines; max 4 mg/day)[1]; 0.1 mg/kg ivi at 2 mg/min (or 4 mg iv)[2].

☠ Beware respiratory depression: have flumazenil and O_2 (± resuscitation trolley) at hand, esp if respiratory disease or giving high doses im/iv. ☠

LOSARTAN/COZAAR
Angiotensin II antagonist: specifically blocks renin–angiotensin system ∴ does not inhibit bradykinin and ⇒ dry cough.
Use: HTN, Px of type 2 DM nephropathy (if ACE-i not tolerated*).
CI: **P/B**.
Caution: RAS, HOCM, mitral/aortic stenosis, **L/R/E**.
SE/Interactions: as captopril, but ↓dry cough (major reason for ACE-i intolerance*). As with ACE-i, can ⇒ ↑K^+ (esp if taking ↑K^+-sparing diuretics/salt substitutes or if RF).
Dose: initially 25–50 mg od (↑ing to max 100 mg od).

☠ Beware if on other drugs that ↑K^+, e.g. amiloride, spironolactone, triamterene, ACE-i and ciclosporin. Don't give with oral K^+ supplements (inc dietary salt substitutes). ☠

LOSEC see Omeprazole; PPI (ulcer-healing drug)

LUGOL'S SOLUTION

Oral I_2 solution.

Use: $\uparrow T_4$ if severe ('thyroid storm' see pp. 206–7) or pre-operatively.

CI: B.

Caution: not for long-term Rx, **P**.

SE: hypersensitivity.

Dose: 0.1–0.3 ml tds (of solution containing 130 mg iodine/ml).

MADOPAR see Co-beneldopa; L-dopa for Parkinson's

MAGNESIUM SULPHATE (iv)

Mg^{++} replacement.

Use: life-threatening asthma[1], serious arrhythmias[2] (esp if torsades or if $\downarrow K^+$; often caused by $\downarrow Mg^{++}$), MI[3] (equivocal evidence of $\downarrow$mortality), eclampsia/pre-eclampsia[4] ($\downarrow$s seizures), symptomatic $\downarrow Mg^{++}$[5] (mostly 2° to GI loss).

Caution: monitor BP, respiratory rate and urine output, **L/R**.

SE: flushing, $\downarrow$BP, GI upset, thirst, $\downarrow$reflexes, weakness, confusion/drowsiness. Rarely arrhythmias, respiratory depression, coma.

Interactions: $\uparrow$risk of $\downarrow$BP with Ca^{2+} channel blockers.

Dose: 4–8 mmol iv over 20 min[1]; 8 mmol iv over 10–15 min[2] (repeating once if required); 8 mmol iv over 20 min then ivi of 65–72 mmol over 24 h[3]; see SPC/BNF[4]; up to 160 mmol iv/im according to need[5] (over up to 5 days). For iv injection, use concentrations of $\leq$20%; if using 50% solution dilute 1 part with $\geq$1.5 parts water for injection.

MANNITOL

Osmotic diuretic.

Use: cerebral oedema[1] (and glaucoma).

CI: pulmonary oedema, **H**.

SE: GI upset, fever/chills, oedema. Rarely seizures, HF.

Dose: 1 g/kg (= 5 ml/kg of 20% solution) as rapid ivi[1].

MAXOLON see Metoclopramide; antiemetic (DA antagonist)

MEBEVERINE
Antispasmodic: direct action on GI muscle.
Use: GI smooth-muscle cramps (esp IBS, diverticulitis).
CI: ileus (paralytic).
Caution: porphyria, P.
SE: hypersensitivity/skin reactions.
Dose: 135–150 mg tds (20 min before food) or 200 mg bd of SR preparation (Colofac MR).

MEFENAMIC ACID/PONSTAN
Mild NSAID; unselective COX inhibitor.
Use: musculoskeletal pain (esp dysmenorrhoea), menorrhagia.
CI/Caution/SE/Interactions: as ibuprofen, but also CI if IBD, caution if porphyria and can ⇒ severe diarrhoea, skin reactions, blood disorders (esp haemolytic ↓Hb, ↓Pt) ∴ stop drug if suspect. mild **W+**.
Dose: 500 mg tds po.

MEFLOQUINE/LARIAM
Antimalarial; kills asexual forms of *Plasmodium*
Use: malaria Px[1] (in areas of chloroquine-resistant falciparum spp) and rarely as Rx *if not taking the drug as Px*.
CI: hypersensitivity *to mefloquine or quinine*, Hx of neuro-Ψ disorders (inc depression, convulsions).
Caution: epilepsy, cardiac conduction disorders, L/P/B.
SE: GI upset, neuro-Ψ reactions (dizziness, ↓balance, headache, convulsions, sleep disorders, neuropathies, tremor, anxiety, depression, psychosis, hallucinations, panic attacks, agitation). Also cardiac fx (AV block, other conduction disorders, ↑ or ↓HR, ↑ or ↓BP), hypersensitivity reactions.
Warn: can ↓driving/other skilled tasks and ⇒ neuro-Ψ reactions.
Interactions: ↑risk of seizures with quinine, chloroquine and hydroxychloroquine. ↓s fx of anticonvulsants (esp valproate and carbamazepine). ↑risk of arrhythmias with amiodarone, quinidine, moxifloxacin and pimozide. Avoid artemether/lumefantrine.

Dose: 250 mg once-weekly[1] (↓dose if Wt <45 kg)$^{SPC/BNF}$.

Need to start Px 2½ wks before entering endemic area (to identify neuro-ψ reactions; 75% of reactions occur by 3rd dose) and continue for 4 wks after leaving endemic area.

MESALAZINE

'New' aminosalicylate: as sulfasalazine, but with ↓sulphonamide SEs.
Use: UC (Rx/maintenance of remission).
CI: *hypersensitivity to any salicylates,* coagulopathies, **R** (caution only if mild), **L** (caution only if not severe).
Caution: P/B/E.
SE: **GI upset, blood disorders**, hypersensitivity (inc **lupus**), RF.
Warn: report unexplained bleeding, bruising, fever, sore throat or malaise.
Monitor: U&E, FBC (stop drug if blood disorder suspected).
Interactions: fx ↓by lactulose. NSAIDs and azathioprine may ↑nephrotoxicity.
Dose: as Asacol (or Ipocol, Pentasa or Salofalk).

MESNA

Binds to metabolite (acreolin) of thiol-containing chemotherapy agents (cyclophosphamide, ifosfamide, oxazaphosphorines), which are toxic to urothelium and can ⇒ severe haemorrhagic cystitis. Give as Px before chemotherapy; see SPC for details.

METFORMIN

Oral antidiabetic (biguanide): ⇒ ↑insulin sensitivity w/o affecting levels (⇒ ↓gluconeogenesis and ↓GI absorption of glucose and ↑peripheral use of glucose). Only active in presence of endogenous insulin (i.e. functional islet cells).
Use: type 2 DM: usually 1st-line if diet control unsuccessful (esp if obese, as ⇒ less ↑Wt than sulphonylureas). Rarely for PCOS.
CI: DKA, ↑risk of lactic acidosis† (e.g. severe dehydration/infection/peripheral vascular disease, shock, major trauma, respiratory failure, alcohol dependence, **recent MI***, general anaesthetic** or iodine-containing radiology contrast media***), **L/R/P/B**.

SE: GI upset (esp initially or if ↑doses), metallic taste, headache. Rarely ↓vitamin B_{12} absorption, lactic acidosis[†] (stop drug).
Dose: initially 500 mg mane, ↑ing as required to max 3 g/day usually in 2 or 3 divided doses. *Take with meals.*

☠ *Both often coexist in coronary angiography: stop drug on day of procedure (giving insulin if necessary; see pp. 167–70) and restart 48 h later, having checked that renal function has not deteriorated. Stop on day of surgery ahead of general anaesthetic** and restart when renal function normal. ☠

METHADONE

Opioid agonist: ↓euphoria and long $t_{1/2}$ (⇒ ↓withdrawal symptoms) compared with other opioids.
Use: opioid dependence as aid to withdrawal.
CI/Caution/SE/Interactions: as Morphine but levels not ↑by ritonavir, but are by voriconazole and cimetidine.
Dose: *individual requirements vary widely according to level of previous abuse:* sensible starting dose is 10–20 mg/day po, ↑ing by 10–20 mg every day until no signs or symptoms of withdrawal – which usually stop at 40–60 mg/day. Then aim to wean off gradually. Available as non-proprietary solutions (1 mg/ml) or as Methadose (10 mg/ml or 20 mg/ml). Can give sc/im[SPC/BNF].

☠ Do not confuse solutions of different strengths. ☠

METHIONINE

Sulphur-containing amino acid: binds toxic metabolites of paracetamol.
Use: paracetamol OD *<12 h post-ingestion* (ineffective after this), mostly when acetylcysteine ivi cannot be given (e.g. outside hospital).
CI: metabolic acidosis.
Caution: schizophrenia (can worsen), L.
SE: N&V, irritability, drowsiness.
Interactions: can ↓fx of L-dopa.
Dose: 2.5 g po 4-hourly (for *4 doses only: total dose = 10 g*).

METHOTREXATE

Immunosuppressant, antimetabolite: dihydrofolate reductase inhibitor (↓s nucleic acid synthesis).

Use: rheumatoid arthritis[1] (1st-line DMARD), **psoriasis** (if severe/resistant), **Ca** (ALL, non-Hodgkin's lymphoma, choriocarcinoma, various solid tumours), rarely in Crohn's disease.

CI: severe blood disorders, active infections, immunodeficiency, **R/L** (if either significant, otherwise caution), **P** (females and *males* must avoid conception for ⩾3 months after stopping treatment), **B**.

Caution: effusions (esp ascites and pleural effusions: accumulates and returns to blood ⇒ ↑toxicity), blood disorders, UC, PU, ↓immunity, porphyria, **E**.

SE: mucositis/GI upset, myelosuppression, skin reactions. Rarely **pulmonary fibrosis/ pneumonitis** (esp in rheumatoid arthritis), hepatotoxicity, neurotoxicity (inc necrotising demyelinating leukoencephalopathy), seizures, RF (esp tubular necrosis).

Monitor: U&Es, FBC, LFTs.

Interactions: NSAIDs*, trimethoprim, co-trimoxazole, corticosteroids, probenecid, nitrous oxide, pyrimethamine, clozapine, cisplatin, acitretin, ciclosporin all ⇒ ↑toxicity ± levels.

Warn: avoid over-the-counter NSAIDs*, report any clinical features of infection (esp sore throat).

Dose: 7.5 mg **once a week**[1] (can split dose into 3 × 2.5 mg at 12-h intervals), max 20 mg/wk. For other uses see BNF/SPC.

☠NB: dose is only once a week: potentially fatal if given daily. ☠

METHOTRIMEPRAZINE see Levomepromazine; DA antagonist.

METHYLDOPA

Centrally acting α_2 agonist.

Use: HTN; esp pregnancy-induced and 1° HTN during pregnancy.

CI: depression, phaeo, porphyria, **L** (inc active liver disease).

Caution: Hx of depression/liver impairment, **R**.

SE: (minimal if dose <1 g/day) dry mouth, sedation, dizziness, weakness, headache, GI upset, postural ↓BP, ↓HR. Rarely **blood disorders, hepatotoxicity**, pancreatitis, Ψ disorders, parkinsonism.

Monitor: FBC, LFTs.

Interactions: ↑s neurotoxicity of lithium. Hypotensive fx ↑d by antidepressants, anaesthetics and salbutamol ivi. ☠**MAOIs**.☠

Dose: initially 250 mg bd/tds (125 mg bd in elderly), ↑ing gradually at intervals ≥2 days (max 2g/day in elderly) to max of 3 g/day.

METHYLPREDNISOLONE

Glucocorticoid (mild mineralocorticoid activity).

Use: acute flares of inflammatory diseases[1] (esp rheumatoid arthritis, MS), cerebral oedema, Rx of graft rejection.

CI/Caution/SE/Interactions: see Steroids section (pp. 185–7).

Dose: acutely, up to 1 g ivi od[1] (normally for 3 days). Also available po and as im depot.

METOCLOPRAMIDE/MAXOLON

Antiemetic: D_2 antagonist: acts on central chemoreceptor trigger zone and directly stimulates GI tract (⇒ ↑motility).

Use: N&V, esp GI (gastroduodenal, biliary, hepatic) or opiate-/chemotherapy-induced.

CI: GI obstruction/perforation/haemorrhage (inc 3–4 days post-GI surgery), phaeo, **B**.

Caution: epilepsy, porphyria, L/R/P/E.

SE: extrapyramidal fx (see p. 192 – esp in elderly and young females: reversible if drug stopped w/in 24 h or with procyclidine), **drowsiness**, restlessness, GI upset, behavioural/mood Δs, ↑prolactin. Rarely skin reactions, neuroleptic malignant syndrome.

Interactions: ↑s fx of NSAIDs and ciclosporin levels. ↑s risk of extrapyramidal fx of antipsychotics, SSRIs and TCAs.

Dose: 10 mg tds po/im/iv.

METOLAZONE

Potent thiazide-like diuretic: as bendroflumethiazide, plus has additive diuretic fx with loop diuretics.

Use: oedema[1], HTN[2].

CI/Caution/SE/Interactions: see Bendroflumethiazide.

Dose: 5–10 mg od po (mane), ↑ing if needed to max of 80 mg/day[1]; initially 5 mg od, then on alternate days for maintenance[2].

METOPROLOL

β-blocker, cardioselective ($\beta_1 > \beta_2$), short-acting.
Use: HTN[1], angina[2], arrhythmias[3], migraine Px[4], ↑T_4 (adjunct)[5].
CI/Caution/SE/Interactions: see Propranolol.
Dose: 50–100 mg bd po[1,4]; 50–100 mg bd/tds po[2,3]; 50 mg qds po[5].
Can give iv[SPC/BNF]. See p. 197 for use in AMI/ACS.

METRONIDAZOLE/FLAGYL

Antibiotic, 'cidal': binds DNA of anaerobic (and microaerophilic)
bacteria/protozoa.
Use: anaerobic and protozoal infections, abdominal sepsis (esp
bacteroides), aspiration pneumonia, *C. difficile* (AAC), *H. pylori*
eradication (see p. 145), giardia/entamoeba infections, Px during GI
surgery. Also dental/gynaecological infections, bacterial vaginosis
(*Gardnerella*), PID.
Caution: avoid with alcohol: drug metabolised to acetaldehyde
and other toxins ⇒ flushing, abdominal pain, ↓BP (= 'disulfiram-
like' reaction), porphyria, **L/P/B**.
SE: GI upset (esp N&V), metallic taste, skin reactions. Rarely,
drowsiness, headache, dizziness, dark urine, hepatotoxicity, blood
disorders, myalgia, arthralgia, seizures (transient), ataxia,
peripheral neuropathy (if prolonged Rx).
Interactions: can ↑lithium/phenytoin levels, **W+**.
Dose: 500 mg tds po/iv for severe infections. Lower doses can
be given po (using 200-mg or 400-mg tablets) or higher doses pr
(1 g bd/tds) according to indication[SPC/BNF].

MICONAZOLE/DAKTARIN

Imidazole antifungal (topical) but *systemic absorption can occur*.
Use: oral fungal infections.
CI: L.
Caution: porphyria, **P/B**.
SE: GI upset. Rarely hypersensitivity, hepatotoxicity.
Interactions: as ketoconazole, but less commonly significant. **W+**.
Dose: oral gel 5–10 ml qds (after food).

L/R/H = **L**iver, **R**enal and **H**eart failure (full key see p. viii)

MIDAZOLAM

Benzodiazepine, very short-acting (see p. 190).

Use: sedation for stressful/painful procedures (esp if amnesia desirable).

CI/Caution/SE/Warn/Interactions: see Diazepam, plus can ↑fx of ciclosporin and nifedipine.

Dose: 1.0–7.5 mg iv; initially 2 mg (1 mg if elderly) over 30 secs, then titrate up slowly until desired sedation achieved using 0.5–1.0-mg boluses over 30 secs. Can aslo give im[SPC/BNF].

☠ Beware respiratory depression: have flumazenil and O_2 (± resuscitation trolley) at hand, esp if respiratory disease or giving high doses im/iv. ☠

MINOCYCLINE

Tetracycline antibiotic: inhibits ribosomal (30S subunit) protein synthesis; broadest spectrum of tetracyclines.

Use: acne[1].

CI/Caution/SE/Interactions: as tetracycline, but ↓bacterial resistance, although ↑risk of SLE and irreversible skin/body fluid discoloration. Can also use (with caution) in RF.

Dose: 100 mg bd po[1] (can ↑to bd for other indications).

MINOXIDIL

Peripheral vasodilator (arterioles ≫ veins): also ⇒ ↑CO, ↑HR, fluid retention ∴ *always needs concurrent β-blocker and diuretic*.

Use: HTN (if severe and Rx-resistant).

CI: phaeo.

Caution: IHD, porphyria, R/P/B.

SE: hypertrichosis, coarsening of facial features (reversible, but makes it *unsuitable for women*), ↑Wt, peripheral oedema, pericardial effusions, angina (dt ↑HR). Rarely, GI upset, gynaecomastia/breast tenderness, renal impairment, skin reactions.

Dose: initially 2.5–5 mg/day in 1 or 2 divided doses, ↑ing if needed up to max of 50 mg/day (↓dose in elderly and dialysis patients). Also used topically for male-pattern baldness.

MIRTAZAPINE/ZISPIN
Antidepressant: **N**oradrenaline **A**nd **S**pecific **S**erotonin **A**gonist (NASSA); specifically stimulates $5HT_1$ receptors (antagonises $5HT_2/5HT_3$), antagonises central presynaptic α_2 receptors.
Use: depression, esp in elderly* or if insomnia†.
CI/Caution/SE: as fluoxetine, but ⇒ ↓**sexual dysfunction**/GI upset, ↑**sedation**† (esp during titration) and ↑appetite/Wt (can be beneficial in elderly*). Rarely, blood disorders (inc agranulocytosis**), Δ LFTs, convulsions, myoclonus, oedema.
Warn: patient to report signs of infection** (esp sore throat, fever): stop drug and check FBC if concerned.
Interactions: avoid with other sedatives (inc alcohol), sibutramine and artemether/lumefantrine. ☠Never give with MAOIs.☠
Dose: initially 15 mg nocte (max 45 mg/day).

MISOPROSTOL
PGE_1 analogue: ↓s gastric secretions.
Use: Rx/Px of PU (esp NSAID-induced). Also unlicensed use for induction of medical abortion and ripening cervix for surgical abortion.
CI: ☠**pregnancy**☠ (actual or planned), **B**.
Caution: cardiovascular/cerebrovascular disease.
SE: diarrhoea. Rarely, other GI upset, menstrual Δs, uterine pains.
Dose: most often used with diclofenac as Arthrotec. (Also available with naproxen as Naprotec.)

MIXTARD "biphasic" insulin preparations, available as 20, 30, 40 or 50, which refer to the percentage of soluble (short-acting) insulin; the rest is isophane (long-lasting) insulin.

MMF see Mycophenolate mofetil; immunosuppressant

MOEXIPRIL/PERDIX
ACE-inhibitor for HTN
CI/Caution/SE/Monitor/Interactions: see Captopril.
Dose: initially 7.5 mg od (3.75 mg if taking diuretics/nifedipine, elderly, LF or RF) ↑ing according to response to max 30 mg/day.

MONTELUKAST/SINGULAIR

Leukotriene receptor antagonist: ↓s Ag-induced bronchoconstriction.
Use: *non-acute* asthma (see BTS guidelines, p. 152), esp if large exercise-induced component.
Caution: acute asthma, Churg-Strauss syndrome P/B.
SE: headache, GI upset, myalgia, dry mouth/thirst. Rarely
Churg–Strauss syndrome: asthma (± rhin-/sinus-itis) with systemic vasculitis and ↑EØ*.
Monitor: FBC* and for development of vasculitic (purpuric/non-blanching) rash, peripheral neuropathy, ↑respiratory/cardiac symptoms: all signs of possible Churg–Strauss syndrome.
Dose: 10 mg nocte (↓doses if <14 years old$^{SPC/BNF}$).

MORCAP SR CAPSULES morphine tablets (20, 50 or 100 mg).
Doses given od/bd; see palliative care section (p. 158).

MORPHGESIC SR morphine tablets (10, 30, 60 or 100 mg). Doses given bd; see palliative care section (p. 158).

MORPHINE

Opioid analgesic.
Use: severe pain (inc post-op), AMI and acute LVF.
CI: acute respiratory depression, ↑risk of paralytic ileus, acute alcoholism, ↑ICP/head injury (respiratory depression ⇒ CO_2 retention and cerebral vasodilation ⇒ ↑ICP), phaeo.
Caution: ↓respiratory reserve (esp asthma, COPD), ↓BP, ↓T_4, ↑prostate, convulsive disorders, pancreatitis, biliary tract disorders, L (can ⇒ **coma**: avoid using or give minimum dose), R/P/B/E.
SE: N&V, respiratory depression, constipation* (can ⇒ **ileus**), seizures (at ↑doses), ↓BP (rarely ↑BP), sedation, dry mouth, urinary retention, biliary tract spasms, anorexia, mood Δ (↑ or ↓), ↓libido, **dependence**. Rarely, skin reactions, ↓Pt.
Interactions: ☠MAOIs (don't give within 2 wks of).☠ Levels ↑by ritonavir. ↑s fx of other CNS depressants (esp SSRIs and TCAs).
Dose: 5–15 mg sc/im up to 4-hourly; 2.5–10 mg iv up to 4-hourly (at 2 mg/min). NB: iv doses are generally ¼–½ that of im doses.

Can ↑dose and frequency with expert supervision and always adjust dose to response (in chronic pain, can use po as Oramorph, MST, Morphgesic, Morcap, MXL, Sevredol or Zomorph see p. 158). *Unless short-term Rx, always consider laxative Px**.

☠If ↓BMI or elderly, titrate dose up slowly, monitor O$_2$ sats and have naloxone ± resuscitation trolley at hand.☠

MST CONTINUS SR oral morphine. Need to specify if *tablets* (5, 10, 15, 30, 60, 100 or 200 mg) or *suspension* (sachets of 20, 30, 60, 100 or 200 mg to be mixed with water). Doses given bd; see Palliative care section (p. 158).

MUPIROCIN/BACTROBAN
Topical antibiotic for bacterial infections (esp nasal MRSA); available as ointment and cream (*specify which*) bd/tds.

Local MRSA eradication protocols often exist; if not, then a sensible regimen is to give for 5–10 days and then swab 2 days later, repeating regimen if culture still positive.

MXL CAPSULES morphine capsules (30, 60, 90, 120, 150 or 200 mg). Doses given od; see Palliative care section (p. 158).

MYCOPHENOLATE MOFETIL (MMF)
Immunosuppressant: ↓s B-/T-cell lymphocytes (and ↓s Ab production by B-cells).
Use: transplant rejection Px, autoimmune diseases, vasculitis.
CI: P/B
Caution: active serious GI diseases[†], **E**.
Monitor: FBC (4-wkly for 2 months, then monthly for 1st yr).
Warn: patient to report unexplained bruises/bleeding/signs of infection. Avoid strong sunlight*.
SE: GI upset, blood disorders (esp ↓NØ, ↓Pt), weakness, tremor, headache, ↑cholesterol, ↑ or ↓K$^+$. Rarely GI ulceration/bleeding/ perforation[†], hepatotoxicity, skin neoplasms*.
Interactions: ↑risk of agranulocytosis with clozapine.
Dose: *Specialist use only*[SPC/BNF].

N-ACETYLCYSTEINE see Acetylcysteine; paracetamol antidote.

NALOXONE
Opioid receptor antagonist for opiate reversal if OD or over-Rx.
Caution: Cardiovascular disease, cardiotoxic drugs, H.
Dose: 0.4–2.0 mg iv (or sc/im), repeating after 2 min if no response
(or ↑ing if severe poisoning). *Short-acting*: often needs repeating
every 2–3 min (max total 10 mg) and consider ivi (10 mg made up to
50 ml with 5% dextrose; useful start rate is 60% of initial dose over
1 h, then adjusted to response).

NALTREXONE
Opioid antagonist: ↓s euphoria of opioids if dependence and ↓s
craving and relapse rate in alcoholic withdrawal (opioids thought to
mediate alcohol addiction; not licensed for this in UK yet).
Use: Opioid and alcohol withdrawal; start >1 wk after stopping*.
CI: if still taking opioids (can precipitate withdrawal*), **L** (inc acute
hepatitis).
Caution: R/P/B.
SE: GI upset, **hepatoxicity**, sleep and ψ disorders.
Monitor: LFTs.
Dose: initial dose 25 mg od po, thereafter 50 mg od (or 250 mg per
week split into 2 × 100 mg and 1 × 150 mg doses); specialist
use only.
NB: also ↓s fx of opioid analgesics.

NAPROXEN
NSAID (propionic acid derivative): unselective COX inhibitor.
Use: arthritis[1], acute musculoskeletal pain[2] (esp
post-orthopaedic surgery), acute gout[3], dysmenorrhoea[4].
CI/Caution/SE/Interactions: as ibuprofen, but ↑SEs (esp GI).
Dose: 250–500 mg bd[1]; 500 mg initially then 250 mg 6–8-hourly[2,4];
750 mg initially then 250 mg 8-hourly[3]. Also available with
misoprostol as Px against PU (as Napratec).

NARCAN see Naloxone

NICORANDIL

K^+-channel activator ($\Rightarrow$ arterial dilation $\Rightarrow$ $\downarrow$afterload) with nitrate component ($\Rightarrow$ venous dilation $\Rightarrow$ $\downarrow$preload).

Use: angina Px/Rx (unresponsive to other Rx).

CI: $\downarrow$BP (esp cardiogenic shock), LVF with $\downarrow$filling pressures.

Caution: hypovolaemia, acute pulmonary oedema, P/B.

SE: headache (often only initially*), **flushing**, dizziness, weakness, N&V, $\downarrow$BP, $\uparrow$HR (dose-dependent). Rarely, oral ulcers, myalgia, angioedema, hepatotoxicity.

Interactions: ☠ risk of $\downarrow\downarrow$BP with sildenafil, tadalafil and vardenafil. ☠

Dose: 5–30 mg bd (start low, esp if susceptible to headaches*).

NIFEDIPINE

Ca^{2+} channel blocker (dihydropyridine): dilates smooth muscle, esp arteries (inc coronaries). Reflex sympathetic drive $\Rightarrow$ $\uparrow$HR and $\uparrow$contractility $\therefore$ $\Rightarrow$ $\downarrow$HF cf other Ca^{2+} channel blockers (e.g. verapamil, and to a lesser degree diltiazem), which $\Rightarrow$ $\downarrow$HR + $\downarrow$contractility. Also diuretic fx*.

Use: angina Px[1], HTN[2], Raynaud's[3].

CI: cardiogenic shock, clinically significant aortic stenosis, ACS (inc w/in 1 month of MI), porphyria.

Caution: angina or LVF can worsen (consider stopping drug), $\downarrow$BP, DM, L ($\downarrow$dose), R/H/P/B.

SE: flushing, headache, ankle oedema, dizziness, $\downarrow$BP, palpitations, rash/pruritus, GI upset, weakness, myalgia, arthralgia. Rarely, PU, hepatotoxicity and poly-/noct-uria.

Interactions: metab by **P450**. $\uparrow$ fx of digoxin. $\downarrow$s fx of quinidine. Ciclosporin and grapefruit juice $\uparrow$ fx of nifedipine. Rifampicin, phenytoin and carbamazepine $\downarrow$ fx of nifedipine. Risk of $\downarrow\downarrow$BP with Mg^{++} iv/im.

Dose: 5–20 mg tds po[3]; use long-acting preparations for HTN/ angina, as normal-release preparations $\Rightarrow$ erratic BP control and reflex $\uparrow$HR, which can worsen IHD (e.g. Adalat LA or Retard and many others with differing fx and doses[SPC/BNF]).

NITROFURANTOIN

Antibiotic: 'static' at ↓doses, 'cidal' at ↑doses. Only active in urine (no systemic antibacterial fx).

Use: UTIs.

CI: G6PD deficiency, porphyria, **R** (also ⇒ ↓activity of drug: it needs to be concentrated in urine), **P/B**.

Caution: DM, lung disease, ↓Hb, ↓vitamin B, ↓folate, electrolyte imbalance, susceptibility to peripheral neuropathy, L/E.

SE: GI upset, pulmonary reactions (inc effusions, fibrosis), **peripheral neuropathy, hypersensitivity**. Rarely, hepatotoxicity, cholestasis, pancreatitis, arthralgia, alopecia (transient), skin reactions (esp exfoliative dermatitis), blood disorders, BIH.

Dose: 50 mg qds po (↑to 100 mg if severe chronic recurrent infection); od nocte if for Px. *Take with food.* Not available iv or im.

NB: can ⇒ false positive urine dipstick for glucose and discolour urine.

NORADRENALINE (= NOREPINEPHRINE)

Vasoconstrictor sympathomimetic: stimulates α-receptors ⇒ vasoconstriction.

Use: ↓BP (unresponsive to other Rx)[1], cardiac arrest[2].

CI: ↑BP, **P**.

Caution: thrombosis (coronary/mesenteric/peripheral), Prinzmetal's angina, post-MI, ↑T_4, DM, ↓O_2, ↑CO_2, hypovolaemia (uncorrected), E.

SE: vun ↓BF to vital organs (esp kidney). Also headache, ↓HR, arrhythmias, peripheral ischaemia. ↑BP if over-Rx.

Interactions: 💀 risk of arrhythmias with halothane and cyclopropane. 💀 Risk of ↑BP with clonidine, MAOIs and TCAs.

Dose: 80 μg/ml ivi at 0.16–0.33 ml/min[1] (adjust according to response); 0.5–0.75 ml of 200-μg/ml solution iv stat[2]. (💀 NB: *doses given here are for noradrenaline **acid tartrate**, not **base*** 💀).

NUROFEN see Ibuprofen; NB: 'over-the-counter' use can ⇒ poor response to HTN and HF Rx.

NYSTATIN

Polyene antifungal.

Use: candida infections: topically for skin/mucous membranes (esp mouth/vagina); po for GI infections (not absorbed).

SE: GI upset (at ↑doses), skin reactions.

Dose: topically as gel prn; po suspension: 0.5–1 million units qds, usually for 1 wk, for Rx (or 1 million/units od for Px) *after food*.

OLANZAPINE/ZYPREXA

'Atypical' antipsychotic: D_2 and $5HT_2$ (+ mild muscarinic) antagonist.

Use: schizophrenia[NICE], mania, bipolar Px, acute sedation.

CI: glaucoma (angle-closure), **B**. If giving im also AMI/ACS, ↓↓BP/HR, SSS or recent heart surgery.

Caution: drugs that ↑QTc, dementia, cardiovascular disease (esp if Hx of or ↑risk of CVA/TIA), DM*, ↑prostate, Parkinson's, Hx of epilepsy, blood disorders, paralytic ileus. ↑s fx of alcohol, L/R/H/P/E.

SE: sedation, ↑Wt, ankle oedema, Δ LFTs, postural ↓BP (esp initially ∴ titrate up dose slowly). ↑glucose (rarely ☠DM/DKA☠). Also extrapyramidal/anticholinergic fx (often transient) and rarely neuroleptic malignant syndrome and hepatotoxicity.

Monitor: BG (± HbA_{1C}), LFTs, U & Es, FBC, prolactin, Wt, lipids (and CK if neuroleptic malignant syndrome suspected). If giving im closely monitor cardiorespiratory function.

Interactions: metab by **P450** ∴ many, but most importantly, levels ↓ by carbamazepine and smoking. ↑risk of ↓ NØ with valproate. Levels may be ↑by ciprofloxacin.

Dose: 5–20 mg po daily (pref nocte to avoid daytime sedation). Available in 'melt' form if ↓compliance/swallowing (as Velotab). Available in quick-acting im form (▼) for acute sedation; give 5–10 mg (2.5–5 mg in elderly) repeating 2 h later if necessary to max total daily dose, inc po doses, of 20 mg (max 3 injections/day for 3 days). NB: im doses not recommended with im/iv benzodiazepines which should be given ⩾1 h later (if benzodiazepines already given, use with caution and closely monitor cardiorespiratory function).

OLMESARTAN/OLMETEC

Angiotensin II antagonist: see Losartan.
Use: HTN.
CI: cholestasis, **P/B**.
Caution/SE/Interactions: see Losartan.
Dose: initially 10 mg od, ↑ing to max 40 mg (20 mg in elderly).

OMEPRAZOLE/LOSEC

PPI: inhibits H^+/K^+ ATPase of parietal cells $\Rightarrow$ ↓acid secretion.
Use: PU Rx/Px (esp if on NSAIDs), gastro-oesophageal reflux disease (if symptoms severe or complicated by haemorrhage/ulcers/stricture)[NICE]. Also used for *H. pylori* eradication and ZE syndrome.
Caution: can mask symptoms of gastric Ca, L/P/B.
SE: GI upset, headache, dizziness, arthralgia, weakness, skin reactions. Rarely, hepatotoxicity, blood disorders, hypersensitivity.
Interactions: ↓ (and ↑) **P450** ∴ many, most importantly ↑s **phenytoin**, cilostazol, diazepam and digoxin levels. ↓ fx of keto-/itra-conazole and atazanavir, mild **W+**.
Dose: 20 mg od po, ↑ing to 40 mg in severe/resistant cases and ↓ing to 10 mg od for maintenance if symptoms stable; 20 mg bd for *H. pylori* eradication regimens (see p. 145). If unable to take po (e.g. perioperatively, ↓GCS, on ITU), give 40 mg iv od either over 5 min or as ivi.

NB: also specialist use iv for acute bleeds. Usually as 8 mg/h ivi for 72 h if endoscopic evidence of PU (prescribed as divided infusions, as drug is unstable). Contact pharmacy ± GI team for advice on indications and exact dosing regimens.

ONDANSETRON

Antiemetic: $5HT_3$ antagonist: acts on central and GI receptors.
Use: N&V, esp if resistant to other Rx or severe postoperative/chemotherapy-induced.
Caution: GI obstruction (inc subacute), L (unless mild), P/B.
SE: constipation (or diarrhoea), **headache**, sedation, fatigue, dizziness. Rarely seizures, chest pain, ↓BP, Δ LFTs, rash, hypersensitivity.

Interactions: metab by **P450**. Levels ↓by rifampicin, carbamazepine and phenytoin. ↓s fx of tramadol.
Dose: 8 mg bd po; 16 mg od pr; 8 mg 2–8-hourly iv/im. Max 24 mg/day usually (8 mg/day if LF). Can also give as ivi at 1 mg/h for max of 24 h. Exact dose and route depends on indication[SPC/BNF].

ORAMORPH oral morphine solution for severe pain, esp useful for prn or breakthrough pain (see p. 158 for use in palliative care).
Dose: 5–10 mg up to 4-hourly (can ↑dose with specialist advice).
Solution mostly commonly used is 10 mg/5 ml, but can be 30 mg/5 ml or 100 mg/5 ml ∴ *specify strength if prescribing in ml.*

OTOSPORIN ear drops for otitis externa (esp if bacterial infection suspected): contains antibacterials (neomycin, polymyxin B) and hydrocortisone.
Dose: 3 drops tds/qds.

OXYBUTYNIN
Anticholinergic (selective M_3 antagonist); antispasmodic (↓s bladder muscle contractions).
Use: detrusor instability (also neurogenic bladder instability, nocturnal enuresis).
CI: bladder outflow (or GI) obstruction, urinary retention, severe UC/toxic megacolon, glaucoma (narrow angle), MG, **B**.
Caution: ↑prostate, autonomic neuropathy, hiatus hernia (if reflux), ↑T_4, IHD, arrhythmias, porphyria, L/R/H/P/E.
SE: antimuscarinic fx (see p. 191), GI upset, palpitations/↑HR, skin reactions – mostly dose-related and reportedly less severe in MR preparations*.
Dose: initially 2.5–5 mg bd/tds po (↑ing if required to max of 5 mg qds) or as Lyrinel XL* 5–20 mg od.

OXYCODONE (HYDROCHLORIDE)/OXYNORM
Opiate for moderate–severe pain (esp in Palliative care).
CI/Caution/SE/Interactions: as morphine, plus avoid in porphyria, L/R (if either severe).

Dose: 5 mg 4–6 hrly po (max usually 400 mg/day). Also available
sc/iv (▼): 5 mg sc up to 4-hrly prn; 1–10 mg iv up to 4-hrly;
7.5 mg/24 h sc infusion adjusted to response. Available in MR form
as OxyContin (5–200 mg bd). *N.B: 2 mg po = 1 mg parenteral.*

OXYTETRACYCLINE
Tetracycline antibiotic: inhibits ribosomal protein synthesis.
Use: acne vulgaris (and rosacea).
CI/Caution/SE/Interactions: as tetracycline, plus caution in
porphyria.
Dose: 250–500 mg qds po 1 h before food or on empty stomach.

PABRINEX
Parenteral (iv or im) vitamins that come as a pair of vials. Vial 1
contains B_1 (thiamine*), B_2 (riboflavin) and B_6 (pyridoxine). Vial 2
contains C (ascorbic acid), nicotinamide and glucose.
Use: Acute vitamin deficiencies (esp thiamine*).
Caution: Rarely ⇒ **anaphylaxis** (esp if given iv too quickly).
*See p. 162 for Wernicke's encephalopathy Px/Rx in alcohol
withdrawal.

PAMIDRONATE
Bisphosphonate: ↓s osteoclastic bone resorption.
Use: ↑Ca^{2+} (esp metastatic: also ↓s pain)[1], Paget's disease[2], myeloma.
CI: P/B.
Caution: Hx of thyroid surgery, L/R/H.
SE: 'flu-like symptoms (inc fever, transient pyrexia), **GI upset** (inc
haemorrhage), **dizziness/somnolence** (warn patient common post-
dose), ↑ (or ↓) **BP**, seizures, musculoskeletal pain, osteonecrosis
(esp in cancer patients; consider dental examination or preventative
Rx), e'lyte Δs (↓**PO_4**, ↓ or ↑K^+, ↑Na^+, ↓Mg^{2+}), RF, blood
disorders.
Monitor: e'lytes, Ca^{2+}, PO_4^-.
Dose: 15–90 mg ivi according to indication (±Ca^{2+} levels[1]); *never
given regularly for sustained periods.*

PANTOPRAZOLE

PPI; as omeprazole, but ↓interactions and can ⇒ ↑TGs.
Dose: 40 mg od po (↓ing to 20 mg maintenance if symptoms allow).
If unable to take po (e.g. perioperatively, ↓GCS, on ITU), can give
40 mg iv over ≥2 min (or as ivi) od. ↑doses if ZE syndrome[SPC/BNF].

PARACETAMOL

Antipyretic (directly influences hypothalamic heat regulation centre),
mild analgesic (inhibits PGE_2 synthesis in CNS ⇒ ↑pain threshold);
unlike NSAIDs, *has no anti-inflammatory fx*.
Use: pyrexia, mild pain.
Caution: alcohol dependence, L (CI if severe liver disease), R.
SE: *all rare*; rash, hypoglycaemia, blood disorders, hepatic (rarely
renal) failure – esp if over-Rx/OD (for Mx, see pp. 211–14).
Interactions: W+ if prolonged regular paracetamol use.
Dose: 0.5–1 g qds po/pr prn (for children, see Calpol).

PAROXETINE/SEROXAT

SSRI antidepressant; as fluoxetine, but ↓$t_{1/2}$.
Use: depression[1], other Ψ disorders (social/generalised anxiety
disorder[1], PTSD[1], panic disorder[2], OCD[3])
CI/Caution/SE/Interactions: as fluoxetine, but ↓frequency of
agitation/insomnia, although ↑frequency of **antimuscarinic fx**
(see p. 191), **extrapyramidal fx** (see p. 192) and **withdrawal fx**[*]
(see p. 192).
Dose: initially 20 mg[1,3] (10 mg[2]) mane, ↑ing if required to max
50 mg[1] or 60 mg[2,3] (40 mg if elderly).
Stop slowly as short $t_{1/2}$ ⇒ ↑risk of withdrawal syndrome.

PARVOLEX see Acetylcysteine; antidote for paracetamol poisoning.

PENICILLAMINE

Chelates copper/lead ⇒ ↑elimination (also acts as DMARD): slow
onset of action (6–12 wks).
Use: Wilson's disease[*], copper/lead poisoning, rheumatoid arthritis
(also autoimmune hepatitis, cystinuria).

CI: SLE, **R** (unless mild when only caution).
Caution: penicillin allergy (can also be penicillamine allergic), **P**.
SE: can worsen **neurological symptoms***, **RF** (esp immune nephritis ⇒ proteinuria*: stop drug if severe), **blood disorders** (↓Pt, ↓NØ, agranulocytosis, aplastic ↓Hb), **rashes** (inc SJS, pemphigus), **taste Δs**, **GI upset** (esp nausea, but ↓s if taken with food). Rarely hepatotoxicity, pancreatitis, autoimmune phenomena: poly-/dermato-myositis, Goodpasture's syndrome, lupus-/myasthenia-like syndromes.
Warn: immediately report sore throat, fever, infection, non-specific illness, unexpected bleeding/bruising, purpura, mouth ulcers or rash.
Monitor: FBC, U&Es, urine dipstick ±24-h collection*.
Interactions: ↑risk of agranulocytosis with clozapine. Absorption ↓by antacids and FeSO₄. Can ↓ levels of digoxin.
Dose: 125–2000 mg daily^SPC/BNF.

Can ⇒ ↓pyridoxine which often needs supplementing. Consider stopping if fever, lymphadenopathy, ↓Pt/NØ, proteinuria or worsening neuro symptoms. Sensitivity occurs in 10%; can restart with prednisolone – get senior advice.

PENICILLIN G see Benzylpenicillin

PENICILLIN V see Phenoxymethylpenicillin

PENTASA see Mesalazine; aminosalicylate for UC, with ↓SEs.

PEPPERMINT OIL
Antispasmodic: direct relaxant of GI smooth muscle.
Use: GI muscle spasm, distension (esp IBS).
SE: perianal irritation, indigestion. Rarely rash or other allergy.
Dose: 1–2 capsules tds, before meals and with water.

PERINDOPRIL/COVERSYL
ACE-inhibitor; see Captopril.
Use: HTN, HF.

CI/Caution/SE/Monitor/Interactions: as Captopril, plus can ⇒ mood/sleep Δs.
Dose: initially 2 mg od (unless for HTN and not elderly, RF or taking diuretic, when can start at 4 mg). ↑ if required to maintenance 4–8 mg od.

PETHIDINE

Opiate analgesic; less potent than morphine but quicker action ⇒ ↑euphoria + ↑abuse/dependence potential ∴ not for chronic use.
Use/CI/Caution/SE: as morphine, but ⇒ ↓constipation, CI in severe RF and ↑risk of hyperpyrexia/CNS toxicity with selegiline.
Dose: 25–100 mg up to 4-hourly im/sc (can give 2-hourly post-operatively); 25–50 mg up to 4-hourly iv. Rarely used po[SPC/BNF].

PHENOBARBITAL (= PHENOBARBITONE)

Barbiturate antiepileptic: potentiates GABA (inhibitory neuro-transmitter), antagonises fx of glutamate (excitatory neurotransmitter).
Use: status epilepticus (SEs and interactions limit other uses).
Caution: respiratory depression, porphyria, L/R/P/B/E.
SE: respiratory depression, sedation, ↓BP, ↓HR, ataxia, skin reactions. Rarely, paradoxical excitement (esp in elderly), blood disorders.
Interactions: ↑P450 ∴ many, most importantly ↓s fx of carbamazepine, Ca^{2+} antagonists, corticosteroids, ciclosporin and OCP. Caution with other sedative drugs (esp benzodiazepines), **W−**.
Dose: total of 10 mg/kg as ivi at 50–100 mg/min (max total 1 g).

PHENOXYMETHYLPENICILLIN (= PENICILLIN V)

as benzylpenicillin (penicillin G) but active orally: used for ENT/skin infections (esp erisipelas), Px of rheumatic fever/*S. pneumoniae* infections (esp post-splenectomy).
Dose: 0.5–1.0 g qds po (≥30 min before food).

PHENTOLAMINE

α-blocker, short-acting.
Use: HTN 2° to phaeo (esp during surgery).

CI: ↓BP, IHD.
Caution: PU/gastritis, asthma, R/P/B/E.
SE: ↓BP, ↑HR, dizziness, weakness, flushing, GI upset, nasal congestion. Rarely, coronary/cerebrovascular occlusion, arrhythmias.
Interactions: see Doxazosin.
Dose: 2–5 mg iv (repeat if necessary).

PHENYTOIN

Antiepileptic: blocks Na^+ channels (stabilises neuronal membranes).
Use: status epilepticus[1], tonic–clonic seizures[2], partial seizures[3].
CI: *if iv* (do not apply if po); sinus ↓HR, Stokes–Adams syndrome, SAN block, 2nd-/3rd-degree HB, porphyria.
Caution: DM, porphyria ↓BP, L/H/P (⇒ cleft lip/palate, congenital heart disease), B.
SE (Acute): *dose-dependent:* **drowsiness** (also confusion/dizziness), **cerebellar fx** (see p. 192), **rash** (common cause of intolerance and rarely ⇒ SJS/TEN), N&V, diplopia, dyskinesia (esp orofacial). *If iv, risk of ↓BP,* **arrhythmias*** (esp ↑QTc), '**purple glove syndrome**' (hand damage distal to injection site), CNS/respiratory depression.
SE (Chronic): gum hypertrophy, coarse facies, hirsutism, acne, ↓folate (⇒ megaloblastic ↓Hb), Dupuytren's, peripheral neuropathy, rickets, osteomalacia. Rarely, blood disorders, hepatotoxicity.
Monitor: FBC**, keep serum levels at 10–20 mg/l (narrow therapeutic index). ☠ If iv, closely monitor BP and ECG* (esp QTc) ☠.
Warn: report immediately any rash, mouth ulcers, sore throat, fever, bruising, bleeding.
Interactions: metab by and ↑s **P450** ∴ many; most importantly ↓s fx of OCP, doxycycline, Ca^{2+} antagonists, ciclosporin, keto-/itra-conazole, quinidine, theophyllines, eplerenone, telithromycin, aripiprazole, mianserin, mirtazepine, paroxetine, TCAs and corticosteroids. Fx ↓by rifampicin, theophyllines, mefloquine, pyrimethamine, antipsychotics, TCAs and St John's wort. Levels ↑by NSAIDs, fluoxetine, mi-/flu-/vori-conazole, trimethoprim, cimetidine, esomeprazole, amiodarone, metronidazole, chloramphenicol, clarithromycin, isoniazid and sulphonamides. Complex interactions with other antiepileptics[SPC/BNF]. **W−** (or rarely **W+**).

Dose: po[2,3], 150–500 mg/day in 1–2 divided doses; **iv**[1], load with 15 mg/kg ivi at max rate of 50 mg/min, then maintenance iv doses of approximately 100 mg tds/qds, adjusting to weight, serum levels and clinical response. If available give iv as *fosphenytoin* (NB: doses differ). ☠Stop drug if ↓WCC** is severe, worsening or symptomatic. ☠

PHOSPHATE ENEMA

Laxative enemas; ⇒ osmotic H_2O retention ⇒ ↑ evacuation.
Use: severe constipation (unresponsive to other Rx).
CI: acute GI disorders.
Caution: if debilitated or neurological disorder, E.
SE: local irritation.
Dose: 1 prn.

PHYLLOCONTIN CONTINUS see Aminophylline (MR)
Dose: initially 1 tablet (225 mg) bd po, then ↑ to 2 tablets bd after 1 wk. (Forte tablets of 350 mg used if smoker/other cause of ↓$t_{1/2}$, e.g. interactions with other drugs; see Theophylline.)

PHYTOMENADIONE

Intravenous vit K_1 for warfarin overdose/poisoning; see pp. 173–4.
Caution: give iv injections slowly. P.

PICOLAX see Bowel preparations
Dose: 1 sachet at 8am and 3pm the day before GI surgery or Ix.

PIOGLITAZONE/ACTOS

Thiazolidinedione (=glitazone) antidiabetic; see Rosiglitazone.
Use/CI/Caution/SE/Monitor: see Rosiglitazone.
Dose: initially 15–30 mg od (max 45 mg od)

PIPERACILLIN

Ureidopenicillin: antipseudomonal.
Use: with tazobactam* (β-lactamase inhibitor) as Tazocin, reserved for severe infections.

CI/Caution/SE/Interactions: see Benzylpenicillin.
Dose: see Tazocin*.

PIRITON see Chlorphenamine; antihistamine for allergies.

PLAVIX see Clopidogrel; anti-Pt agent for Px of IHD (and CVA).

POTASSIUM TABLETS see Kay-cee-L (syrup 1 mmol/ml),
Kloref (effervescent 6.7 mmol/tablet), Sando-K (effervescent
12 mmol/tablet) and Slow-K (MR non-effervescent 8 mmol/tablet,
reserved for when syrup/effervescent preparations are inappropriate;
avoid if ↓swallow).

PRAVASTATIN/LIPOSTAT
HMG-CoA reductase inhibitor: 'statin'; ↓s cholesterol/LDL (and TG).
Use/CI/Caution/SE: see Simvastatin.
Interactions: ↑risk of myositis (± ↑levels) with ☠fibrates☠,
nicotinic acid, ciclosporin and ery-/clari-thromycin. Levels ↓by
colestyramine and colestipol.
Dose: 10–40 mg nocte.

PREDNISOLONE
Glucocorticoid (and mild mineralocorticoid activity).
Use: anti-inflammatory (e.g. rheumatoid arthritis, IBD, asthma,
eczema), immunosuppression (e.g. transplant rejection Px, acute
leukaemias), glucocorticoid replacement (e.g. Addison's disease,
hypopituitarism).
CI: systemic infections (w/o antibiotic cover).
Caution/SE/Interactions: see pp. 185–7.
Warn: carry steroid card (and avoid close contact with people who
have chickenpox/shingles if patient has never had chickenpox).
Dose: usually 2.5–15 mg od po for maintenance. In acute/initial
stages, 20–60 mg od often needed (depends on cause and often
physician preference), e.g. acute asthma (40 mg od), acute COPD
(30 mg od), temporal arteritis (40–60 mg daily). Take with food

($\downarrow$Na$^+$, $\uparrow$K$^+$ diet recommended if on long-term Rx). For others causes, consult SPC/BNF, pharmacy or local specialist relevant to the disease.

☠ Warn patient not to stop tablets suddenly (*can $\Rightarrow$ Addisonian crisis*). Requirements may $\uparrow$ if intercurrent illness/surgery. ☠

PROCHLORPERAZINE/STEMETIL

Antiemetic: DA antagonist (phenothiazine ∴ also antipsychotic, but used rarely for this).

Use: N&V (inc labyrinthine disorders).

CI/Caution/SE/Monitor/Warn/Interactions: as chlorpromazine, but CI are relative and $\Rightarrow$ $\downarrow$sedation. NB: can $\Rightarrow$ **extrapyramidal fx** (esp if elderly/debilitated); see p. 192.

Dose: *po*, acutely 20 mg, then 10 mg 2 h later (5–10 mg bd/tds for Px and labyrinthine disorders); *im*, 12.5 mg, then po doses 6 h later; *pr*, 25 mg then po doses 6 h later (5 mg tds pr for migraine). Available as quick-dissolving 3-mg tablets to be placed under lip (Buccastem); give 1–2 bd.

PROCYCLIDINE

Antimuscarinic: $\downarrow$s cholinergic to dopaminergic ratio in extrapyramidal syndromes $\Rightarrow$ $\downarrow$tremor/rigidity. No fx on bradykinesia (or tardive dyskinesia; may even worsen).

Use: extrapyramidal symptoms (e.g. parkinsonism), esp if drug-induced[1] (e.g. antipsychotics).

CI: urinary retention (if untreated), glaucoma* (angle-closure), GI obstruction.

Caution: cardiovascular disease, $\uparrow$prostate, tardive dyskinesia, L/R/H/P/B/E.

SE: antimuscarinic fx (see p. 191), Ψ disturbances, euphoria (can be drug of abuse), glaucoma*.

Warn: can $\downarrow$ability at driving/skilled tasks.

Dose: 2.5 mg tds po prn[1] ($\uparrow$ if necessary to max of 10 mg tds); 5–10 mg im/iv if acute dystonia or oculogyric crisis.

NB: do not stop suddenly: can $\Rightarrow$ rebound muscarinic fx.

L/R/H = Liver, Renal and Heart failure (full key see p. viii)

PROMETHAZINE
Sedating antihistamine.
Use: insomnia (see p. 189).
CI: CNS depression/coma, MAOI w/in 14 days.
Caution: urinary retention, ↑prostate, glaucoma, epilepsy, IHD, asthma, porphyria, pyloroduodenal obstruction, R (↓dose), L/E/P/B.
SE: antimuscarinic fx, hangover sedation, headache.
Warn: can ↓ability at driving/skilled tasks.
Interactions: ↑s fx of anticholinergics, TCAs and sedatives/hypnotics.
Dose: 25 mg nocte (can ↑dose to 50 mg).

PROPRANOLOL
β-blocker (non-selective): $β_1$ ⇒ ↓HR and ↓contractility, $β_2$ ⇒ vasodilation (and bronchoconstriction and glucose release from liver). Also blocks fx of catecholamines, ↓s renin production, slows SAN/AVN conduction.
Use: HTN[1], IHD (angina Rx[2], MI Px[3]), portal HTN[4] (*may worsen liver function*), essential tremor[5], Px of migraine[6], anxiety[7], ↑T_4 (symptom relief[8], thyroid storm[9]), arrhythmias[8] (inc severe[9]).
CI: asthma/Hx of bronchospasm, peripheral arterial disease (if severe), Prinzmetal's angina, severe ↓HR or ↓BP, SSS, 2nd-/3rd-degree HB, cardiogenic shock, metabolic acidosis, phaeo (unless used specifically with α-blockers), **H** (if uncontrolled).
Caution: COPD, 1st-degree HB, DM*, MG, Hx of hypersensitivity (may ↑ to *all* allergens), L/R/P/B.
SE: ↓HR, ↓BP, HF, peripheral vasoconstriction (⇒ cold extremities, worsening of claudication/Raynaud's), fatigue, depression, sleep disturbance (inc nightmares), hyperglycaemia (and ↓sympathetic response to *hypo*glycaemia*), GI upset. Rarely, conduction/blood disorders.
Interactions: ☠verapamil and diltiazem ⇒ risk of HB and ↓HR ☠. ↓by NSAIDs. ↑s risk of bupivacaine toxicity. ↑s risk of AV block, myocardial depression and ↓HR with amiodarone. Levels of both drugs can ↑with chlorpromazine. Risk of ↑BP with adrenaline and noradrenaline.

Dose: 80–160 mg bd po[1]; 40–120 mg bd po[2]; 40 mg qds for 2–3 days, then 80 mg bd po[3] (start 5–21 days post-MI); 40 mg bd po[4] ($\uparrow$dose if necessary); 40 mg bd/tds po[5,6]; 40 mg od po[7] ($\uparrow$dose to tds if necessary); 10–40 mg tds/qds[8]; 1 mg iv over 1 min[9] (repeating every 2 min if required, to max of 10 mg).

NB: $\downarrow$po dose in LF and $\downarrow$initial dose in RF. Withdraw slowly (esp in angina; as can $\Rightarrow$ rebound worsening of symptoms).

PROPYLTHIOURACIL

Thionamide antithyroid (peroxidase inhibitor): $\downarrow$s I^- $\Rightarrow$ I_2 $\downarrow$s and $\therefore$ $\downarrow T_{3/4}$ production, as carbimazole does, but also $\downarrow$s peripheral T_4 to T_3 conversion. Possible immunosuppressant fx.

Use: $\uparrow T_4$ (2nd-line in the UK; if carbimazole not tolerated).
Caution: L/R, P/B (can cause fetal/neonatal goitre/$\downarrow T_4$ $\therefore$ use min dose and monitor neonatal development closely; 'block-and-replace' regimen $\therefore$ not suitable as high doses used for this).
SE: blood disorders (esp **agranulocytosis**; stop drug if occurs), **skin reactions** (esp urticaria, rarely cutaneous vasculitis/lupus), fever. Rarely hepatotoxicity, nephritis.
Warn: patient to report symptoms of infection (esp sore throat).
Monitor: **FBC**, clotting.
Dose: 200–400 mg od po until euthyroid, then $\downarrow$ to 50–150 mg od.

PROSCAR see Finasteride; antiandrogen for BPH (and baldness).

PROTAMINE (SULPHATE)

Protein (basic) that binds heparin (acidic).
Use: reversal of heparin following over-Rx/OD or after temporary anticoagulation for extracorporeal circuits (e.g. cardiopulmonary bypass, haemodialysis).
Caution: $\uparrow$risk of hypersensitivity reaction if: 1. Vasectomy, 2. Infertile man, 3. Allergy to fish.
SE: $\downarrow$**BP**, $\downarrow$HR, N&V, flushing, dyspnoea. Rarely pulmonary oedema, hypertension, **hypersensitivity reactions**.

L/R/H = Liver, Renal and Heart failure (full key see p. viii)

Dose: 1 mg per 80–100 units of heparin to be reversed as ivi over 10 min. NB: $t_{1/2}$ of iv heparin is short; ↓doses of protamine if giving >15 mins after last iv heparin administration.

Max total dose 50 mg: ☠*high doses can ⇒ anticoagulant fx!*☠

PROZAC see Fluoxetine; SSRI antidepressant.

PULMICORT see Budesonide; inh steroid for asthma. 50, 100, 200 or 400 μg/puff.

PYRAZINAMIDE
Antibiotic: 'cidal' only against intracellular and dividing bacteria (e.g. TB). Good CSF penetration*.
Use: TB Rx (for initial phase, see p. 143), TB meningitis*.
CI: porphyria, **L** (if severe, otherwise caution).
Caution: DM, gout (avoid in acute attacks), **P**.
SE: hepatotoxicity**, ↑**urate**, GI upset (inc N&V), dysuria, interstitial nephritis, **arthr-/my-algia**, sideroblastic ↓Hb, ↓Pt, rash (and photosensitivity).
Monitor: LFTs**.
Dose: up to 2 g daily – exact dose varies according to Wt and whether Rx is 'supervised' or not[SPC/BNF].

PYRIDOSTIGMINE
Anticholinesterase: inhibits cholinesterase at neuromuscular junction ⇒ ↑ACh ⇒ ↑neuromuscular transmission.
Use: myasthenia gravis.
CI: GI/urinary obstruction.
Caution: asthma, recent MI, ↓HR/BP, arrhythmias, vagotonia, ↑T_4, PU, epilepsy, parkinsonism, **R** (consider ↓ing dose), **P/B/E**.
SE: cholinergic fx (see p. 191) – esp if xs Rx/OD, where ↓BP, bronchoconstriction and (confusingly) weakness can also occur (= cholinergic crisis*); ↑**secretions** (sweat/saliva/tears) and miosis are good clues** of xs ACh.
Interactions: fx ↓d by **aminoglycosides** (e.g. gentamicin), **polymixins**, clindamycin, lithium, quinidine, chloroquine, propranolol and procainamide. It ↑s fx of suxamethonium.

Dose: 30–120 mg po up to qds (can ↑to max total daily dose 1.2 g, but best to keep <450 mg to avoid receptor downregulation).

☠️ ↑ing weakness can be due to *cholinergic crisis** as well as MG exacerbation; if unsure which is responsible**, get senior help (esp if ↓respiratory function) before giving Rx, as the wrong choice can be fatal! ☠️

QUINAPRIL/ACCUPRO
ACE-inhibitor for HTN[1] and CCF[2].
CI/Caution/SE/Monitor/Interactions: see Captopril.
Dose: initially 10 mg od (2.5 mg if for CCF or if elderly, on diuretics or RF) ↑ing according to response to max 40 mg[2] or 80 mg[1] daily.

QUININE
Antimalarial: kills bloodborne schizonts.
Use: malaria Rx[1] (esp falciparum), nocturnal leg cramps[2].
CI: optic neuritis, haemoglobinuria, MG*.
Caution: heart conduction dfx (inc AF, HB), G6PD deficiency, P.
SE: **visual Δs** (inc temporary blindness, esp in OD), **tinnitus** (and vertigo/deafness), **GI upset**, **headache**, **rash/flushing**, **hypersensitivity**, confusion, hypoglycaemia**. Rarely blood disorders, ARF, cardiovascular fx (can ⇒ severe ↓BP in OD).
Monitor: blood glucose** and e'lytes (if given iv).
Interactions: ↑s fx of flecainide and digoxin. ↑s risk of arrhythmias with pimozide, moxifloxacin and amiodarone. ↑risk of seizures with mefloquine. Avoid artemether/lumefantrine.
Dose: 200–300 mg nocte po as quinine *sulphate*[2]. For malaria Rx, see pp. 145–6.

RABEPRAZOLE/PARIET
PPI; as omeprazole, but ↓interactions.
Dose: 20 mg od (↓to 10 mg od for maintenance). Max 120 mg/day.

RAMIPRIL/TRITACE
ACE-inhibitor; see Captopril.
Use: HTN[1], HF[2], Px post-MI[3]. Also Px of cardiovascular disease (if age >55 years and at risk)[4].

Cl/Caution/SE/Monitor/Interactions: as captopril.
Dose: initially 1.25 mg od ($\uparrow$ing slowly to max of 10 mg daily)[1,2];
initially 2.5 mg bd then $\uparrow$ to 5.0 mg bd after 2 days[3] (start 3–10 days
post-MI) then maintenance 2.5–5 mg bd; initially 2.5 mg od ($\uparrow$ing
to 10 mg)[4].

RANITIDINE/ZANTAC

H_2 antagonist $\Rightarrow$ $\downarrow$parietal cell H^+ secretion.
Use: PU (Px if on longterm high dose NSAIDs[1], chronic Rx[2], acute
Rx[3]), reflux oesophagitis.
Caution: porphyria, L/R/P/B. ☠ *May mask symptoms of gastric
cancer.* ☠
SE: *all rare:* GI upset (esp diarrhoea), dizziness, confusion, fatigue,
blurred vision, headache, Δ LFTs (rarely hepatitis), rash. Very rarely
arrhythmias (esp if given iv), hypersensitivity, blood disorders.
Dose: initially 150 mg bd po (or 300 mg nocte)[1,2], $\uparrow$ing to
600 mg/day if necessary but try to $\downarrow$ to 150 mg nocte for maintenance;
50 mg tds/qds iv[3] (or im/ivi[SPC/BNF]).

REOPRO see Abciximab; antiplatelet agent for MI/ACS.

RETEPLASE (= r-PA)

Recombinant plasminogen activator: thrombolytic.
Use/Cl/Caution/SE: see Alteplase and pp. 177–80 but only for Rx of
AMI (i.e. not for CVA).
Dose: 10 units as slow iv injection over ≤2 min, repeating after 30 min.
Concurrent unfractionated iv heparin needed for 48 h; see p. 179.

RIFABUTIN

New rifamycin antibiotic; see Rifampicin.
Use: TB: Rx of pulmonary TB[1] and non-tuberculous mycobacterial
disease.[2] Also Px of *M. avium*[3] (if HIV with $\downarrow$CD4).
Cl/Caution/SE/Warn/Monitor/Interactions: see Rifampicin.
Dose: 150–450 mg od[1]; 450–600 mg od[2]; 300 mg od[3].

RIFAMPICIN

Rifamycin antibiotic: 'cidal' $\Rightarrow$ $\downarrow$RNA synthesis.

Use: TB Rx, *N. meningitides* (meningococcal)/*H. influenzae* (type b) meningitis Px. Rarely for *Legionella*/*Brucella*/*Staphylococcus* infections.
CI: jaundice.
Caution: porphyria, L/R/P/B.
SE: hepatotoxicity, GI upset (inc AAC), headache, fever, 'flu-like symptoms (esp if intermittent use), orange/red body secretions*, SOB, blood disorders, skin reactions, shock, ARF.
Warn: of symptoms/signs of liver disease; report jaundice/persistent N&V/malaise immediately. Warn about secretions.*
Monitor: LFTs, FBC (and U&Es if dose >600 mg/day).
Interactions: ↑P450 ∴ many; most importantly ↓s fx of OCP**, carbamazepine, phenytoin, sulphonylureas, rosiglitazone, atovaquone, keto-/flu-/itra-conazole, ampre-/ataza-/indi-/lopi-/nelfi-/saqui-navir, nevirapine, ciclosporin, siro-/tacro-limus, imatinib, corticosteroids, haloperidol, aripiprazole, disopyramide, quinidine, propafenone, eplerenone and Ca^{2+} antagonists. Levels ↑by clari-/ery-thromycin, flu-/itra-/vori-conazole and ampre-/ataza-/rito-navir. **W−**.
Dose: for TB Rx, see p. 143; for other indications see SPC/BNF. (NB: well absorbed po; give iv *only* if ↓swallow.)
Other contraception** needed during Rx.

RIFATER combination preparation of rifampicin, isoniazid and pyrazinamide for 1st 2 months of TB Rx (⟹ ↓bacterial load/ infectiousness until sensitivities known); see p. 143.

RISEDRONATE

Bisphosphonate: ↓s osteoclastic bone resorption.
Use: osteoporosis (Px[1]/Rx[2], esp if postmenopausal or steroid-induced), Paget's disease[3].
CI: ↓Ca^{2+}, **R** (if severe, otherwise caution), **P/B**.
Caution: delayed GI transit/emptying (esp oesophageal abnormalities). Correct Ca^{2+} and other bone/mineral metabolism (e.g. vit D and PTH function) before Rx.
SE: GI upset, bone/joint/muscle pain, headache, rash, HTN. Rarely chest pain, oedema, ↓Wt, apnoea, bronchitis, sinusitis,

glossitis, nocturia, infections (esp UTIs), amblyopia, iritis, dry eyes/corneal lesions, tinnitus.

Warn: take with full glass of water on an empty stomach ≥ 30 min before, and stay upright until, breakfast*.

Interactions: Ca^{2+}-containing products (inc milk) and antacids ($\Rightarrow$ ↓absorption) ∴ separate doses as much as possible from risedronate.

Dose: 5 mg od[1,2] (or 1 × 35-mg tablet/week as Actonel once a week[2]); 30 mg daily for 2 months[3].

RISPERIDONE/RISPERDAL

'Atypical' antipsychotic: similar to olanzapine ($\Rightarrow$ ↓extrapyramidal fx cf 'typical' antipsychotics, esp tardive dyskinesia)

Use: psychosis/schizophrenia (acute and chronic)[NICE], mania.

CI: phenylketonuria (only if Quicklet form used), **B**.

Caution/SE: Similar to olanzapine but $\Rightarrow$ ↓sedation, ↑hypotension (esp initially: ↑dose slowly and consider retitrating if many doses missed), ↓hyperglycaemia and slightly ↑extrapyramidal fx. Also, consider ↓ing dose in LF/RF.

Interactions: levels may be ↓by carbamazepine and ↑by fluoxetine and paroxetine.

Dose: 0.5 mg–8 mg bd po. Also available as liquid or quick dissolving 1 mg/2 mg tablets ("Quicklets") and as long acting im 2 weekly injections ("Consta" ▼) for ↑compliance.

RIVASTIGMINE/EXELON

Acetylcholinesterase inhibitor that acts centrally (crosses BBB): replenishes ACh, which is ↓d in certain dementias.

Use: Alzheimer's disease[NICE].

CI: L (if severe, otherwise caution), **B**.

Caution: conduction defects (esp SSS), PU susceptibility, Hx of COPD/asthma/epilepsy, bladder outflow obstruction, **R/P**.

SE: cholinergic fx (see p. 191), **GI upset** (esp nausea initially), **headache, dizziness**, behavioural/Ψ reactions. Rarely GI haemorrhage, ↓HR, AV block, angina, seizures, rash.

Dose: 1.5 mg bd initially (↑ing slowly to 3–6 mg bd: specialist review needed for clinical response and tolerance).

ROSIGLITAZONE/AVANDIA

Thiazolidinedione (= glitazone) antidiabetic: ↓s peripheral insulin resistance (and, to lesser extent, hepatic gluconeogenesis).

Use: type 2 DM, currently only recommended in combination with a sulphonylurea or, preferably (esp if obese) metformin, after a combination of sulphonylurea + metformin has been given and not resulted in adequate control or been tolerated[NICE].

CI: insulin use (↑risk of HF), **H** (inc Hx of), **L/P/B**.

Caution: cardiovascular disease, **R**.

SE: oedema (esp if HTN/CCF), ↓**Hb**, ↑**Wt**, GI upset (esp diarrhoea), headache, hypoglycaemia (if also taking sulphonylureas), rarely **hepatotoxicity**.

Monitor: LFTs. ☠*Discontinue if jaundice develops.*☠

Interactions: levels ↓by rifampicin and ↑by gemfibrozil.

Dose: 4 mg od (can ↑dose to max 8 mg/day if given with metformin or used on its own).

▼ROSUVASTATIN/CRESTOR

HMG-CoA reductase inhibitor; 'statin' to ↓cholestrol (and TG).

CI: L (if severe, otherwise caution), **R/P/B**.

Use/Caution/SE: see Simvastatin.

Interactions: ↑risk of myositis with ☠**fibrates** and **ciclosporin**☠, and nicotinic acid. Levels ↓by antacids. Mild **W+**.

Dose: initially 10 mg od. If necessary ↑to 20 mg after ≥ 4 wks (if not of Asian origin or risk factors for myopathy/rhabdomyolysis, can ↑to 40 mg after further 4 wks).

(r)tPA = (Recombinant) tissue-type plasminogen activator; see Alteplase

SALBUTAMOL

β_2 agonist, short-acting: dilates bronchial smooth muscle (and endometrium). Also inhibits mast-cell mediator release.

Use: chronic[1] and acute[2] asthma. Rarely ↑K^+ (give nebs prn), premature labour (iv).

Caution: cardiovascular disease (esp arrhythmias*, susceptibility to ↑QTc, HTN), DM (can ⇒ DKA, esp if iv ∴ monitor GBGs), ↑T_4, **P/B**.

SE: *neurological:* **fine tremor**, headache, nervousness, sleep/behavioural Δs (esp in children); *CVS:* $\uparrow$**HR**, palpitations/arrhythmias (esp if iv), $\uparrow$QTc*; *other:* $\downarrow$**K$^+$**, muscle cramps. Rarely hypersensitivity, **paradoxical bronchospasm**.

Monitor: K$^+$ and glucose (esp if $\uparrow$or iv doses).

Interactions: iv salbutamol $\Rightarrow$ $\uparrow$risk of $\downarrow\downarrow$BP with methyldopa.

Dose: 100–200 µg (aerosol) or 200–400 µg (powder) inh prn up to qds[1]; 2.5–5 mg qds 4-hrly neb[2]. If life-threatening (see p. 201), can $\uparrow$nebs up to every 15 min or give as ivi (initially 5 µg/min, then up to 20 µg/min according to response).

SALMETEROL/SEREVENT

Bronchodilator: long-acting β_2 agonist (LABA).

Use: 1st choice add-on for asthma Rx (on top of short-acting β_2 agonist and inh steroids; see BTS guidelines, p. 152). *Not for acute Rx!*

Caution/SE: as salbutamol.

Dose: 50–100 µg bd inh.

SALOFALK see Mesalazine; 'new' aminosalicylate for UC ($\downarrow$SEs).

SANDO-K

Effervescent oral KCl (12 mmol K$^+$/tablet).

Use: $\downarrow$K$^+$.

CI: K$^+$ > 5.0 mmol/l, **R** (if severe, otherwise caution).

Caution: GI ulcer/stricture, hiatus hernia.

SE: N&V, GI ulceration.

Dose: according to serum K$^+$: average 2–4 tablets/day if diet normal ($\downarrow$dose in RF/elderly, $\uparrow$ if established $\downarrow$K$^+$).

SENNA/SENOKOT

Stimulant laxative.

Use: constipation.

CI: GI obstruction.

SE: GI cramps. If chronic use atonic non-functioning colon, $\downarrow$K$^+$.

Dose: 2 tablets nocte.

SEPTRIN see Co-trimoxazole (sulfamethoxazole + trimethoprim).

SERC see Betahistine; histamine analogue for vestibular disorders.

SEROXAT see Paroxetine; SSRI antidepressant.

SERETIDE combination asthma inhaler with possible synergistic action: long-acting β_2 agonist (LABA); salmeterol 50 µg (Accuhaler) or 25 µg (Evohaler) + fluticasone (steroid) in varying quantities (50, 100, 125, 250 or 500 µg/puff).

SERTRALINE/LUSTRAL
SSRI antidepressant; see Fluoxetine.
Use: depression (also PTSD in women and OCD).
CI/Caution/SE/Warn/Interactions: as fluoxetine, but ↓incidence of agitation/insomnia, doesn't ↑carbamazepine/phenytoin levels, but does ↑pimozide levels.
Dose: initially 50 mg od, ↑ing to max daily dose 200 mg (if >100 mg/day, must be divided into at least 2 doses).

SEVELAMER/RENAGEL
PO_4-binding agent; contains no aluminium/Ca^{2+} ∴ no risk of ↑ing their levels (which can occur with other drugs, esp if on dialysis). Also ↓s cholesterol.
Use: ↑PO_4 (if on dialysis).
CI: GI obstruction.
Caution: GI disorders, P/B.
SE: GI upset, ↓ (or ↑) BP, headache.
Dose: initially 800–1600 mg tds po, then adjust according to response.

SEVREDOL oral morphine tablets (10 mg, 20 mg or 50 mg).
Dose: 10–50 mg up to 4-hourly.

SILDENAFIL/VIAGRA or REVATIO (▼)
Phosphodiesterase type 5 inhibitor: ↑s local fx of NO (⇒ ↑smooth-muscle relaxation ∴ ↑blood flow into corpus cavernosum).
Use: erectile dysfunction.

CI: recent CVA/MI/ACS, ↓BP, hereditary degenerative retinal disorders and other conditions where vasodilation/sexual activity inadvisable. **L/H** (if either severe).

Caution: cardiovascular disease, bleeding disorders (inc active PU), anatomical deformation of penis, predisposition to prolonged erection (e.g. multiple myeloma/leukaemias/sickle cell disease), R.

SE: headache, flushing, GI upset, dizziness, visual disturbances, nasal congestion, hypersensitivity reactions. Rarely, serious cardiovascular events, priapism and painful red eyes.

Interactions: 💀 Nitrates (e.g. GTN/ISMN/ISDN/nicorandil) can ↓↓BP ∴ never give together. 💀 Antivirals (esp ritonavir) ↑ its levels.

Dose: initially 50 mg approx 1 h before sexual activity, adjusting to response (1 dose per 24 h, max 100 mg per dose).

SIMVASTATIN/ZOCOR

HMG-CoA reductase inhibitor ('statin'): ⇒ ↓cholesterol (↓s synthesis), ↓LDL (↑s uptake), mildly ↓s TG.

Use: ↑cholesterol, Px of atherosclerotic disease: IHD (inc 1° prevention), CVA, PVD.

CI: porphyria, **L** (inc active liver disease or ΔLFTs), **P/B**.

Caution: ↓T_4, alcohol abuse, Hx of liver disease, **R** (if severe).

SE: hepatitis and **myositis*** (both rare but important), headache, GI upset, rash, hypersensitivity.

Monitor: LFTs (and CK if symptoms develop*).

Interactions: ↑risk of myositis (± ↑levels) with 💀**fibrates**💀, **nefazodone, clari-/ery-/teli-thromycin, itra-/keto-/mi-conazole, ciclosporin, protease inhibitors,** nicotinic acid, amiodarone, verapamil, diltiazem and grapefruit juice. Mild **W+**.

Dose: 5–80 mg nocte (usually start at 10–20 mg[SPC/BNF]).

💀Myositis* can rarely ⇒ **rhabdomyolysis**, esp if ↓T_4, RF (consider ↓doses) or taking drugs that ↑levels/risk of myositis (see above). 💀

SINEMET see Co-careldopa; L-dopa for Parkinson's.

SLOW-K

Slow-release (non-effervescent) oral KCl (8 mmol K^+/tablet).

Use: ↓K⁺ *where liquid/effervescent tablets inappropriate.*
CI/Caution/SE: as Sando-K, plus caution if ↓swallow.
Dose: according to serum K⁺: average 3–6 tablets/day.

SODIUM BICARBONATE iv

Alkalinising agent.
Use: metabolic acidosis; e.g. if RF, DKA, cardiac arrest* (esp if due
to ↑K⁺ or TCAs; also controversial use if pH < 7.1), certain drug
ODs (esp aspirin and TCAs) and rarely for life-threatening ↑K⁺.
SE: paradoxical intracellular acidosis, ↓s O₂ delivery (O₂ saturation
curve shift), ↑Na⁺, ↑serum osmolality.
Dose: *iv:* available in 1.26%, 4.2% and 8.4% solutions; in cardiac
arrests* give 50 mmol (50 ml of 8.4% solution) repeating if
necessary. NB: *specialist use only* – strongly consider getting senior
help before giving.
☠ Toxic if extravasation when given iv (⇒ tissue necrosis). ☠

SODIUM VALPROATE see Valproate; antiepileptic.

SOTALOL

β-blocker (non-selective); class II(+III) antiarrhythmic.
Use: Px of SVT (esp of paroxysmal AF), **Rx of VT** (if life-threatening/
symptomatic, esp non-sustained or spontaneous sustained dt IHD or
cardiomyopathy), Px of ventricular ectopics.
CI: as propranolol, plus ↑QT syndromes, torsades de pointes, **R** (if
severe, otherwise caution and ↓dose).
Caution: as propranolol, plus electrolyte Δs (⇒ ↑risk of
arrhythmias, esp if ↓K⁺/↓Mg²⁺; ∴ beware if severe diarrhoea).
SE: as propranolol, plus arrhythmias (can ⇒ ↑**QT** ± **torsades de
pointes***, esp in females).
Interactions: ☠ *Verapamil and diltiazem ⇒ risk of ↓HR and
HB.* ☠ Disopyramide, quinidine, procainamide, amiodarone, TCAs
and antipsychotics ⇒ ↑**risk arrhythmias***.
Dose: 40–160 mg bd po (↑if life threatening to max 640mg/day);
20–120 mg iv over 10 min (repeat 6-hourly if necessary).
Give under specialist supervision and with ECG monitoring.

▼SPIRIVA see Tiotropium; new inhaled muscarinic antagonist.

SPIRONOLACTONE
K+-sparing diuretic: aldosterone antagonist at distal tubule (also potentiates loop and thiazide diuretics).
Use: ascites (esp 2° to cirrhosis or malignancy), oedema, HF (adjunct to ACE-i and/or another diuretic), nephrotic syndrome, 1° aldosteronism.
CI: ↑K+, ↓Na+, Addison's, **P/B**.
Caution: porphyria, **L/R/E**.
SE: ↑K+, **gynaecomastia**, GI upset (inc N&V), impotence, ↓BP, ↑Na+, rash, confusion, headache, hepatotoxicity, blood disorders.
Monitor: U&E.
Interactions: ↑s digoxin and lithium levels. ↑s risk of RF with NSAIDs (which also antagonise its diuretic fx).
Dose: 100–400 mg/day po (25 mg od if for HF).
☠Beware if on other drugs that ↑K+, e.g. amiloride, triamterene, ACE-i, angiotensin II antagonists and ciclosporin. Do not give with oral K+ supplements inc dietary salt substitutes. ☠

STEMETIL see Prochlorperazine; DA antagonist antiemetic.

STREPTOKINASE
Thrombolytic agent: ↑s plasminogen conversion to plasmin ⇒ ↑fibrin breakdown.
Use: AMI, TE of arteries (inc PE, central retinal artery) or veins (DVT, central retinal vein).
CI/Caution/SE: see pp. 177–80.
Dose: AMI: 1.5 million units ivi over 60 min; **other indications:** 250 000 units ivi over 30 min, then 100 000 units ivi every hour for up to 12–72 h (see SPC).

STREPTOMYCIN
Aminoglycoside antibiotic.
Use: TB (if isoniazid resistance established before Rx); see p. 143.
CI/Caution/SE/Interactions: see Gentamicin.

SULFASALAZINE

Aminosalicylate: combination of the immune modulator
5-aminosalicylic acid (5-ASA) and the antibacterial sulfapyridine
(a sulphonamide).

Use: rheumatoid arthritis[1]. Also UC[2] (inc maintenance of remission)
and active Crohn's disease[2], but not 1st-line, as newer drugs
(e.g. mesalazine) have ↓ sulphonamide SEs; still used if well-
controlled with this drug and with no SEs or if joint manifestations.

CI: sulphonamide or salicylate hypersensitivity, **R** (caution if mild).

Caution: slow acetylators, Hx of any allergy, porphyria, G6PD
deficiency, **L/P/B**.

SE: GI upset (esp ↓appetite/Wt), **hepatotoxicity**, **blood disorders**,
hypersensitivity (inc severe skin reactions), seizures, lupus.

Monitor: LFTs, U&Es, FBC.

Dose: 500 mg/day ↑ing to max 3 g/day[1]; 1–2 g qds po for acute
attacks[2], ↓ing to maintenance of 500 mg qds – can also give 0.5–1.0 g
pr bd after motion (as supps) ± po Rx or 3 g pr nocte (as enema).

SYMBICORT combination asthma inhaler: each puff contains
long-acting $β_2$ agonist (LABA) formoterol 4.5 µg + steroid
budesonide 80 µg (as '100/6' preparation), 160 µg (as '200/6'
preparation) or 320 µg (as '400/12' preparation).

SYNACTHEN = SYNthetic ACTH (adrenocorticotrophic hormone)

Use: Dx of Addison's disease; in 'short' test will find ↓plasma
cortisol 0, 30 and 60 mins after 250 µg iv/im dose.

CI: allergic disorders (esp asthma). NB: can ⇒ anaphylaxis.

TACROLIMUS (= FK 506)

Immunosuppressant (calcineurin inhibitor): ↓s IL-2-mediated
LØ proliferation.

Use: Px of transplant rejection (esp renal).

CI: macrolide hypersensitivity, **P** (exclude before starting), **B**.

Caution/SE: as ciclosporin, but ⇒ ↑neuro-/nephro-toxicity
(although ⇒ ↓hypertrichosis/hirsutism); also **diabetogenic** and
rarely ⇒ cardiomyopathy.

Interactions: metab by **P450** ∴ many, but most importantly: ↑s levels of ☠ciclosporin☠. Levels ↑by clari-/ery-/teli-thromycin, chloramphenicol, antifungals, ataza-/rito-/nelfi-navir, nifedipine and diltiazem. Levels ↓by rifampicin and St John's wort. Nephrotoxicity ↑by NSAIDs, gentamicin and amphotericin. Avoid with other drugs that ↑K⁺.

Dose: specialist use^SPC/BNF.

Interactions important: ↑levels ⇒ toxicity; ↓levels may ⇒ rejection.

▼TADALAFIL/CIALIS

Phosphodiesterase type-5 inhibitor; see Sildenafil.

CI: recent CVA/MI/ACS, ↓BP, uncontrolled HTN/arrhythmias and other conditions where vasodilation/sexual activity inadvisable. **L** (if severe), **H**.

Use/Caution/SE/Interactions: as sildenafil plus ⇒ ↓↓BP with α-blockers.

Dose: initially 10 mg ≥ 30 min before sexual activity, adjusting to response (1 dose per 24 h, max 20 mg per dose).

TAMOXIFEN

Oestrogen receptor antagonist.

Use: oestrogen receptor-positive Ca breast[1] (as adjuvant Rx: ⇒ ↑survival, delays metastasis), anovulatory infertility[2].

CI: **P** (*exclude before starting Rx*).

Caution: ↑risk of TE* (if taking cytotoxics), porphyria, B.

SE: hot flushes, GI upset, menstrual/endometrial Δs (☠inc Ca: if Δ vaginal bleeding/discharge or pelvic pain/pressure ⇒ urgent Ix☠). Also fluid retention, exac of bony metastases pain. Many other gynaecological/blood/skin/metabolic Δs (esp lipids, LFTs).

Warn: of symptoms of endometrial cancer and TE* (and to report calf pain/sudden SOB).

Interactions: **W+**.

Dose: 20 mg od po[1]; for anovulatory infertility[2] see SPC/BNF.

TAMSULOSIN/FLOMAX MR*

α₁ blocker ⇒ internal urethral sphincter relaxation (∴ ⇒ ↑bladder outflow) and systemic vasodilation.

Use: BPH.
CI/Caution/SE/Interactions: as Doxazosin plus **L** (if severe).
Dose: 400 μg mane (after food). Available in MR preparation*.

TAZOCIN combination of piperacillin (antipseudomonal penicillin) + tazobactam (β-lactamase inhibitor).
Use: severe infections/sepsis (mostly in ITU setting or if resistant to other antibiotics).
CI/Caution/SE/Interactions: as Benzylpenicillin.
Dose: 2.25–4.5 g tds/qds iv.

TEGRETOL see Carbamazepine; antiepileptic.

TEICOPLANIN

Glycopeptide antibiotic; 'cidal' against aerobes and anaerobes.
Use: serious Gram-positive infections (mostly reserved for MRSA).
Caution: vancomycin sensitivity, R/P/B.
SE: GI upset, hypersensitivity/skin reactions, blood disorders, nephrotoxicity, ototoxicity (but less than vancomycin), ΔLFTs, local reactions at injection site.
Monitor: U&Es, LFTs, FBC, auditory function (esp if chronic Rx or on other oto-/nephro-toxic drugs, e.g. gentamicin, amphotericin B, ciclosporin, cisplatin and furosemide).
Dose: single loading dose of 400 mg im/iv, then ↓ to 200 mg od 24 h later (if severe infection continue at 400 mg 12-hourly for 2 more doses before changing to 200 mg od; if life threatening then change to 400 mg od). ↑dose if weight >85 kg, severe burns or endocarditis and ↓dose if RF; see SPC.

TELMISARTAN/MICARDIS

Angiotensin II antagonist; see Losartan.
Use: HTN.
CI: biliary obstruction, **L** (if severe, otherwise caution), **P/B**.
Caution/SE/Interactions: as Losartan, plus ↑s digoxin levels.
Dose: 20–80 mg od (usually 40 mg od).

TEMAZEPAM

Benzodiazepine, short-acting.
Use: insomnia.
CI/Caution/SE/Interactions: see Diazepam.
Dose: 10 mg nocte (can ↑dose if tolerant to benzodiazepines, but beware respiratory depression). *Dependency common:* max 4-wk Rx.

TENECTEPLASE (= TNK-tPA)/METALYSE

Recombinant thrombolytic; advantageous as given as single bolus.
Use: Acute myocardial infarction.
CI/Caution/SE: see pp. 177–80.
Dose: iv bolus over 10 s according to weight: ≥90 kg, 50 mg; 80–89 kg, 45 mg; 70–79 kg, 40 mg; 60–69 kg, 35 mg; <60 kg, 30 mg. Concurrent unfractionated iv heparin needed for 24–48 h; see p. 179.

TERAZOSIN/HYTRIN

α₁ blocker ⇒ internal urethral sphincter relaxation (∴ → ↑bladder outflow) and systemic vasodilation.
Use: BPH (and rarely HTN).
Caution: Hx of micturition syncope or postural ↓BP, P/B.
SE/Interactions: see Doxazosin. '1st-dose collapse' common.
Dose: initially 1 mg nocte, ↑ing as necessary (max 20 mg/day).

TERBINAFINE/LAMISIL

Antifungal: oral[1,2] or topical cream[3].
Use: ringworm[1] (Tinea spp), dermatophyte nail infections[2], fungal skin infections[3].
Caution: psoriasis (may worsen), autoimmune disease (risk of lupus-like syndrome), L/R/P/B (only P/B apply if giving topically).
SE: headache, GI upset, mild rash, joint/muscle pains. Rarely neuro-Ψ disturbances, blood disorders, hepatic dysfunction, serious skin reactions (stop drug if progressive rash).
Dose: 250 mg od po for 2–6 wks[1] or 6 wks – 3 months[2]; 1–2 topical applications/day for 1–2 wks.

TERBUTALINE/BRICANYL

Inhaled β_2 agonist similar to salbutamol.

Dose: 250–500 µg od–qds inh (powder or aerosol); 5–10 mg up to qds neb. Can also give po/sc/im/iv[SPC/BNF].

TETRACYCLINE

Tetracycline broad-spectrum antibiotic: inhibits ribosomal (30S subunit) protein synthesis.

Use: acne vulgaris[1] (or rosacea), genital/tropical infections (doxycycline often preferred).

CI: age <12 years (**stains/deforms teeth**), **R/P/B**.

Caution: may worsen MG or SLE, **L**.

SE: GI upset (rarely AAC), oesophageal irritation, headache, dysphagia. Rarely hepatotoxicity, blood disorders, photosensitivity, hypersensitivity, visual Δs (rarely 2° to BIH; stop drug if suspected).

Interactions: ↓absorption with milk (do not drink 1 h before or 2 h after drug), antacids and Fe/Al/Ca/Mg/Zn salts. ↓s fx of OCP (small risk). ↑risk of BIH with retinoids. Mild **W+**.

Dose: 500 mg bd po[1], otherwise 250–500 mg tds/qds po.

NB: take >30 min before food.

THEOPHYLLINE

Methylxanthine bronchodilator. *Theories of action:* 1. ↑s intracellular cAMP; 2. adenosine antagonist; 3. ↓s diaphragm fatigue. NB: additive fx with β_2 agonists (but with ↑risk of SEs, esp ↓K⁺).

Use: severe asthma/COPD: acute (iv as aminophylline; see pp. 201–2) or chronic (po; see p. 152 for BTS asthma guidelines).

CI: hypersensitivity to any 'xanthine' (e.g. aminophylline/theophylline), acute porphyria.

Caution: cardiac disease (risk of arrhythmias*), epilepsy, ↑T_4, PU, HTN, fever, porphyria, acute febrile illness, glaucoma, DM, **L/P/B/E**.

SE: (tachy)**arrhythmias***, seizures (esp if given rapidly iv), **GI upset** (esp **nausea**), CNS stimulation (restlessness, insomnia), headache, ↓K⁺.

Monitor: K⁺, serum levels (pre and post dose) as narrow therapeutic window (10–20 mg/l = 55–110 µmol/l) but toxic fx can occur even in this range.

Interactions: P450 ($\Rightarrow$ very variable $t_{1/2}$): **levels ↑d in** HF/liver disease/viral infections/elderly, and if taking **fluvoxamine**/cimetidine/ ciprofloxacin/ macrolides (ery-/clari-thromycin)/propranolol/'flu vaccines/fluc-/keto-conazole/OCP/diltiazem/verapamil. **Levels ↓d in** smokers/chronic alcohol abuse, and if taking phenytoin/ carbamazepine/phenobarbital/rifampicin/ritonavir/St John's wort.
Dose: 125–250 mg tds/qds po (MR preparations often preferred, as ↓SE; 4 brands available, all different doses[SPC/BNF]). NB: available iv as aminophylline.

THIAMINE (= vitamin B$_1$)
Use: replacement for nutritional deficiencies (esp in alcoholism).
Dose: 100 mg tds po in severe deficiency (25 mg od if mild/chronic). For iv preparations, see Pabrinex and pp. 161–3 for Mx of acute alcohol withdrawal.

THYROXINE (= LEVOTHYROXINE)
Synthetic T_4 (NB: thyroxine often now called 'levothyroxine').
Use: ↓T_4 Rx (for maintenance); NB: acutely, liothyronine (T_3) often needed – see p. 207.
CI: ↑T_4.
Caution: panhypopituitarism/other predisposition to adrenal insufficiency (*corticosteroids needed first*), chronic ↓T_4, cardio-vascular disorders (esp HTN/IHD; can worsen)*, DI, DM**, P/B/E.
SE: features of ↑T_4 (should be minimal unless xs Rx): D&V, tremors, restlessness, headache, flushing, sweating, heat intolerance, angina, arrhythmias, palpitations, ↑HR, muscle cramps/weakness, ↓Wt. Also osteoporosis (esp if xs dose given; use min dose necessary).
Interactions: can Δ digoxin and antidiabetic** requirements, can ↑fx of TCAs and ↓levels of propranolol. **W+.**
Dose: 25–200 μg mane (titrate up slowly, esp if elderly/HTN/IHD*).

TINZAPARIN/INNOHEP
Low-molecular-weight heparin.
Use: DVT/PE Rx[1] and Px[2] (inc preoperative). Not licensed for MI/unstable angina (unlike other LMWHs).

CI/Caution/SE/Monitor/Interactions: as Heparin, plus CI if breastfeeding (**B**) and caution in asthma ($\Rightarrow$ ↑hypersensitivity reactions).
Dose: (all sc) 175 units/kg od[1]; 50 units/kg or 4500 units od[2] (3500 units od if low risk).

Consider monitoring anti Xa (3–4 h post dose) if RF (i.e. creatinine > 150), pregnancy, Wt >100 kg or <45 kg; see p. 175.

▼TIOTROPIUM/SPIRIVA

New long-acting inh muscarinic antagonist for asthma; similar to ipratropium, but only for chronic use and caution in RF.
Dose: 18 µg od inh.

TIROFIBAN/AGGRASTAT

Antiplatelet agent: glycoprotein IIb/IIIa receptor inhibitor – stops binding of fibrinogen and inhibits platelet aggregation.
Use: Px of MI in unstable angina/NSTEMI (*if last episode of chest pain w/in 12 h*), esp if high risk and awaiting PCI[NICE] (see p. 198).
CI: abnormal bleeding or CVA w/in 30 days, haemorrhagic diathesis, Hx of haemorrhagic CVA, intracranial disease (neoplasm/aneurysm/AVM), severe HTN, ↓Pt, ↑INR **B**.
Caution: ↑risk of bleeding (e.g. drugs, recent bleeding/trauma/procedures; see SPC/BNF), **L** (avoid if severe), **H** (if severe), **R/P**.
SE: bleeding, nausea, fever, ↓Pt (reversible).
Monitor: FBC (baseline, 2–6 h after giving, then at least daily).
Dose: 400 *nanograms*/kg/min for 30 min, then 100 *nanograms*/kg/min for ≥48 h (continue for 12–24 h post-PCI), for max of 108 h. Needs concurrent heparin.

Specialist use only: get senior advice or contact on-call cardiology.

TOLBUTAMIDE

Oral antidiabetic (short-acting sulphonylurea).
Use/CI/Caution/SE/Interactions: as glibenclamide, but shorter action and hepatic metabolism* means ↓risk of hypoglycaemia, esp in elderly/RF* (↓reliance on renal excretion). Can also $\Rightarrow$ headache.
Dose: 0.5–2.0 g daily in divided doses, with food.

TOLTERODINE/DETRUSITOL

Antimuscarinic, antispasmodic.
Use: detrusor instability; urinary incontinence/frequency/urgency.
CI/Caution/SE: as oxybutynin (mostly antimuscarinic fx;
see p. 191), **P/B**.
Dose: 1–2 mg bd po. (MR preparation available as 4 mg od po; not
suitable if RF or LF).

tPA (= tissue-type Plasminogen Activator) see Alteplase.

TRAMADOL

Opioid analgesic: also ↓s pain by ↑ing 5HT/adrenergic transmission.
Use: moderate pain (esp musculoskeletal).
CI/Caution/SE/Interactions: as morphine, but ↓respiratory
depression, ↓constipation, ↓addiction. Rarely ⇒ Ψ disturbances.
Also **P/B** and **W+**.

Dose: 50–100 mg up to 4-hourly po (or im/iv) to max 400 mg/day.
Postoperatively; initially 100 mg im/iv, then 50 mg every 10–20 min
to max total dose of 250 mg in 1st h, then prn (max 600 mg/day).

TRANDOLAPRIL/GOPTEN OR ODRIK

ACE-inhibitor for HTN, HF and LVF post-MI.
CI/Caution/SE/Monitor/Interactions: see Captopril.
Dose: initially 0.5 mg od, ↑ing at intervals of 2–4 wks if required to
max 4 mg od. ↓doses if given with diuretic. If for LVF post MI,
start ≥3 days after MI.

TRANEXAMIC ACID

Antifibrinolytic: competitively inhibits activation of plasminogen
to plasmin.
Use: bleeding: acute bleeds[1] (esp 2° to anticoagulants, thrombolytic/
anti-Pt agents, epistaxis, haemophilia), menorrhagia[2], hereditary
angioedema[3].
CI: TE disease, **R** (if severe, otherwise caution).

Caution: gross haematuria (can clot and obstruct ureters), DIC, P.
SE: GI upset, colour vision Δs (stop drug), TE.
Dose: 15–25 mg/kg bd/tds po (if severe, 0.5–1 g tds iv)[1]; 1 g tds po
for 4 days (max 4 g/day)[2]; 1–1.5 g bd/tds[3].

TRIAMTERENE

K^+-sparing diuretic (weak).
Action/Use/CI/Caution/SE: as amiloride, but ⇒ less ↓BP ∴ not
used for HTN (unless used with other drugs).
Warn: urine may go blue.
Interactions: ↑s lithium levels. NSAIDs ↑risk of RF and ↑K^+.
Dose: almost exclusively used with stronger K^+-wasting diuretics
in combination preparations (e.g. co-triamterzide). For use alone,
initially give 150–250 mg daily, ↓ing to alternate days after 1 wk.
☠Beware if on other drugs that ↑K^+, e.g. amiloride, spironolactone, ACE-i, angiotensin II antagonists and ciclosporin. Do not
give with oral K^+ tablets or dietary salt substitutes. ☠

TRI-IODOTHYRONINE

See Liothyronine; synthetic T_3 mostly used in myxoedema coma.

TRIMETHOPRIM

Antifolate antibiotic ('static'): inhibits dihydrofolate reductase.
Use: UTIs (rarely other infections).
CI: blood disorders (esp megaloblastic ↓Hb).
Caution: ↓folate (or predisposition to), porphyria, R/P/B/E.
SE: see Co-trimoxazole (Septrin), but much less frequent and severe
(esp BM suppression, skin reactions). Also **GI upset**, rash, rarely
other hypersensitivity.
Warn: those on long-term Rx to look for signs of blood disorder
and to report fever, sore throat, rash, mouth ulcers, bruising or
bleeding.
Interactions: ↑s phenytoin levels. ↑s risk of arrhythmias with
amiodarone, antifolate fx with pyrimethamine and toxicity with
ciclosporin, azathioprine, mercaptopurine and methotrexate. **W+.**

L/R/H = Liver, Renal and Heart failure (full key see p. viii)

Dose: 200 mg bd po (100 mg nocte for chronic infections or as Px if at risk; NB: risk of ↓folate if long-term Rx).

TROPICAMIDE EYE DROPS

Antimuscarinic: mydriatic (short-acting, weak), cycloplegic.
Use: eye examination.
CI: glaucoma (angle closure).
Caution: ↑IOP (inc predisposition to), inflamed eye (↑risk of systemic absorption).
SE: blurred vision, ↓accommodation. Rarely precipitation of glaucoma (↑risk if >60 yrs and long sighted).
Dose: 1–2 drops 0.5 or 1.0% solution 15–20 min before examination.

TURBOHALER inh delivery device for asthma drugs.

(SODIUM) VALPROATE

Antiepileptic and mood stabiliser: potentiates and ↑s levels of inhibitory neuropeptide GABA.
Use: epilepsy[1], mania and off licence for other Ψ disorders.
CI: porphyria, personal or family Hx of severe liver dysfunction, **L** (inc active liver disease).
Caution: SLE, ↑bleeding risk*, R, P (⇒neural-tube/craniofacial dfx), B.
SE: sedation, cerebellar fx (see p. 193; esp tremor, ataxia), headache, GI upset, ↑Wt, SOA, alopecia, skin reactions, ↓cognitive/motor function, Ψ disorders, encephalopathy (2° to ↑NH_4). Rarely but seriously **hepatotoxicity, blood disorders** (esp ↓Plt*), **pancreatitis** (mostly in 1st 6 months of Rx).
Warn: of clinical features of pancreatitis and liver/blood disorders. Inform women of childbearing age of teratogenicity/need for contraception.
Monitor: LFTs, FBC ± serum levels *pre-dose* (therapeutic range 50–100 mg/l; useful for checking compliance but ↓use for efficacy).
Interactions: fx ↓d by antimalarials (esp mefloquine), antidepressants, antipsychotics and some antiepileptics[SPC/BNF]. Levels ↓by cimetidine. ↑s fx of aspirin and primidone. ↑risk of ↓NØ with olanzapine. Mild **W+**.

Dose: initially 300 mg bd, ↑ing to max of 2.5 g/day[1].
Can give false-positive urine dipstick for ketones.

VALSARTAN/DIOVAN

Angiotensin II antagonist; see Losartan.
Use: HTN[1], MI with LV failure/dysfunction[2].
CI: biliary obstruction, cirrhosis, **L** (if severe)/**P/B**.
Caution/SE/Interactions: see Losartan.
Dose: initially 80 mg od[1] (40 mg if >75 yrs old, LF, RF or
↓intravascular volume) or 20 mg bd[2], ↑ing if necessary to max
160 mg od[1]/bd[2].

VANCOMYCIN

Glycopeptide antibiotic. Poor po absorption (unless bowel
inflammation*), but still effective against C. *difficile*** as acts
'topically' in GI tract.
Use: serious Gram-positive infections[1] (inc endocarditis Px and
systemic MRSA), AAC[2] (give po).
Caution: Hx of deafness, IBD* (only if given po), **R/P/B/E**.
SE: nephrotoxicity, ototoxicity (stop if tinnitus develops), **blood
disorders, rash, hypersensitivity** (inc anaphylaxis, severe skin
reactions), nausea, fever, phlebitis/irritation at injection site. Also
shock or rash/flushing of upper body if given too rapidly iv.
Monitor: serum levels: keep predose trough levels 5–10 mg/l; start
monitoring after 3rd dose (1st dose if RF). Also U&Es, FBC,
urinalysis (and auditory function if elderly/RF).
Interactions: ↑nephrotoxicity with ciclosporin. ↑ototoxicity with
loop diuretics. ↑s fx of suxamethonium.
Dose: 1 g bd ivi over 100 min[1] (↓dose in elderly); 125 mg qds po[2].

▼VARDENAFIL/LEVITRA

Phosphodiesterase type-5 inhibitor; see Sildenafil.
Use/CI/Caution/SE/Interactions: as sildenafil plus caution if
susceptible to (or taking durgs that) ↑QTc, can ⇒ ↓↓BP with
α-blockers and levels ↑by keto-/itra-conazole and grapefruit juice.

Dose: initially 10 mg (5 mg if elderly) approx 25–60 min before sexual activity, adjusting to response (1 dose per 24 h, max 20 mg per dose).

VENLAFAXINE/EFEXOR

Serotonin and **N**oradrenaline **R**euptake **I**nhibitor (SNRI): antidepressant with ↓ sedative/antimuscarinic fx cf TCAs. ↑danger in OD/heart disease than other antidepressants.

Use: depression (2nd line[NICE])[1], generalised anxiety disorder.

CI: conditions with ↑ arrhythmia risk, uncontrolled HTN, **H** (if severe), **P/B**.

Caution: heart disease, Hx of mania, seizures or glaucoma. **L/R**.

SE: GI upset, ↑BP (dose-related; monitor BP if dose >200 mg/day), **withdrawal fx** (see p. 192 common even if doses only a few hours late), **rash** (consider stopping drug, as can be 1st sign of severe reaction*), insomnia/agitation, dry mouth, sexual dysfunction, drowsiness, dizziness, headache.

Warn: report rashes* and can ↓driving/skilled task ability.

Interactions: ☠ *Never give with MAOIs.* ☠ metab by **P450**; levels ↑by ketoconazole & erythromycin. ↑s risk of bleeding with aspirin/NSAIDs and CNS toxicity with selegiline/sibutramine. Avoid artemether/lumefantrine. ↑s levels of clozapine. Mild **W+**.

Dose: 37.5–187.5 mg bd po[1]; start low and ↑ dose if required. Efexor XL MR od preparation available (max 225 mg od).

MHRA advises specialist supervision for initiation if severely depressed, hospitalised or dose ≥300 mg/day.

VENTOLIN see Salbutamol; β_2 agonist bronchodilator.

VERAPAMIL

Ca^{2+} channel blocker (rate-limiting type): fx on heart (⇒ ↓HR, ↓contractility*) > vasculature (dilates peripheral/coronary arteries); i.e. reverse of the dihydropyridine type (e.g. nifedipine). Only Ca^{2+} channel blocker w useful antiarrhythmic properties (class IV).

Use: HTN[1], angina[2], arrhythmias (SVTs, esp instead of adenosine if asthma)[3].

CI: ↓BP, ↓HR (<50 bpm), 2nd-/3rd-degree HB, SAN block, SSS, AF or atrial flutter 2° to WPW, porphyria. **H*** (inc Hx of).

Caution: AMI, 1st degree HB, L/P/B.

SE: constipation (rarely other GI upset), **HF**, ↓**BP** (dose-dependent), HB, headache, dizziness, fatigue, ankle oedema, hypersensitivity, skin reactions.

Interactions: ↑risk of AV block and HF with ☠ β-blockers ☠ disopyramide, flecainide and amiodarone. ↑s hypotensive fx of antihypertensives (esp α-blockers) and anaesthetics. ↑s fx of digoxin, theophyllines, carbamazepine and ciclosporin. Rifampicin ↓s its fx. ↓s levels of quinidine. ↑risk of myopathy with simvastatin. Sirolimus ↑s levels of both drugs. Risk of VF with ☠ iv dantrolene ☠.

Warn: fx ↑d by grapefruit juice (avoid).

Dose: 80–160 mg tds po[1]; 80–120 mg tds po[2]; 40–120 mg tds po[3]; 5–10 mg iv (over ≥2 min with ECG monitoring), followed by additional 5 mg iv if necessary after 5–10 min[3].

VIAGRA see Sildenafil; phosphodiesterase inhibitor.

VITAMIN K see Phytomenadione

VOLTAROL see Diclofenac; moderate-strength NSAID.

WARFARIN

Oral anticoagulant: blocks synthesis of vitamin-K-dependent factors (II, VII, IX, X) and proteins C and S.

Use: Rx/Px of TE; see pp. 171–4.

CI: severe HTN, PU, bacterial endocarditis, **P**.

Caution: recent surgery, L/R/B.

SE: haemorrhage, rash, fever, diarrhoea. Rarely other GI upset, 'purple-toe syndrome', skin necrosis, hepatotoxicity, hypersensitivity.

Warn: fx are ↑d by alcohol and cranberry juice (avoid).

Dose: see pp. 171–4.

☠ NB: **W+** and **W−** denote significant interactions throughout this book: take particular care with antibiotics and drugs that affect cytochrome **P450** (see p. 193). ☠

XALATAN see Latanoprost; topical PG analogue for glaucoma.

ZANTAC see Ranitidine; H_2 antagonist.

ZAFIRLUKAST/ACCOLATE
Leukotriene receptor antagonist; ↓s Ag-induced bronchoconstriction.
Use: asthma (non-acute).
CI: cirrhosis, **L/B**.
Caution: Churg–Strauss syndrome, **R/P/E**.
SE/Monitor: as Montelukast, but ↑**hepatotoxicity**, **W+**.
Dose: 20 mg bd po.

ZALEPLON
'Non-benzodiazepine' hypnotic; see Zopiclone.
Use/CI/Caution/SE/Interactions: see Zopiclone.
Dose: 10 mg nocte (5 mg if elderly).

ZESTRIL see Lisinopril; ACE-i.

ZIDOVUDINE (AZT)
Antiviral (nucleoside analogue): reverse-transcriptase inhibitor.
Use: HIV Rx (and Px, esp of vertical transmission).
CI: severe ↓NØ or ↓Hb (caution if other blood disorders), **B**.
Caution: ↓B_{12}, ↑ risk of lactic acidosis, **L/R/P/E**.
SE: blood disorders (esp ↓Hb or ↓WCC), **GI upset**, **headache**,
fever, taste Δs, sleep disorders. Rarely hepatic/pancreatic
dysfunction, myopathy, seizures, other neurological/Ψ disorders.
Interactions: Levels ↑by fluconazole. fx ↓by ritonavir.
↑myelosuppression with ganciclovir. ↓s fx of stavudine.
Dose: see SPC/BNF.

ZIRTEK see Cetirizine; non-sedating antihistamine for allergies.

▼ZOLEDRONIC ACID/ZOMETA
Bisophosphonate: ↓s osteoclastic bone resorption.
Use: Px of bone damage[1] or Rx of ↑Ca^{2+} in malignancy[2].
CI: P/B.
Caution: cardiac disease, dehydration*, ↓Ca^{2+}/PO_4^{2-}/Mg^{2+}. **R** (↓dose).

SE: 'flu-like syndrome, fever, bone pain, fatigue, N&V. Also arthr-/my-algia, $\downarrow Ca^{2+}/PO_4^{2-}/Mg^{2+}$, pruritis/rash, headache, conjunctivitis, RF, hypersensitivity, blood disorders (esp $\downarrow$Hb) and **osteonecrosis** (esp of jaw; consider dental examination or preventive Rx).

Monitor: Ca^{2+}, PO_4^{2-}, Mg^{2+}. Check U&E plus adequately hydrated pre-dose*.

Interactions: Ca^{2+}-containing products (inc milk) and antacids ($\Rightarrow \downarrow$absorption) $\therefore$ separate doses as much as possible from risedronate.

Dose: 4 mg ivi every 3–4 weeks[1]; 4 mg ivi as single dose[2].

ZOLPIDEM

'Non-benzodiazepine' hypnotic; see Zopiclone.
Use/CI/Caution/SE/Interactions: see Zopiclone.
Dose: 10 mg nocte (5 mg if elderly).

ZOMORPH Morphine tablets (10, 30, 60, 100 or 200 mg). Doses given bd; see Palliative care section p. 158.

ZOPICLONE

Short-acting hypnotic (cyclopyrrolone): potentiates GABA pathways via same receptors as benzodiazepines (although isn't a benzodiazepine!): can also $\Rightarrow$ dependence* and tolerance.

Use: insomnia (not long-term*).
CI: respiratory failure, sleep apnoea, MG, **L** (if severe**), **P/B**.
Caution: Ψ disorders, Hx of drug abuse*, **R/E**.
SE: *all rare:* GI upset, taste Δs, behavioural/Ψ disturbances (inc psychosis, aggression), hypersensitivity.
Interactions: Levels $\uparrow$by ritonavir.
Dose: 7.5 mg nocte, $\uparrow$ing to 12.5 mg if necessary. If LF (non-severe**), RF or elderly give 3.75 mg.

ZOTON see Lansoprazole; PPI.

▼ZYBAN see Buproprion; adjunct to smoking cessation.

Drug selection

ANTIBIOTICS

IMPORTANT POINTS

- The following *are only guides to a rational start to Rx*. Local organisms, sensitivities and prescribing preferences vary widely: if unsure, consult your microbiology department/pharmacy.
- Empirical ('best guess') Rx is given unless stated otherwise.
- When deciding if 'severe' treatment is necessary, consider each individual's comorbidity and if you have time to give simple Rx first and then add on or change if patient is not improving.
- Get as many appropriate cultures as possible *before* starting Rx; if unfamiliar with patient, check for recent culture results to aid choice of agent.

> It is essential to ask each patient *in person* about allergies before prescribing any antibiotics. Do not rely on notes or drug charts, which are often not complete or accurate. Remember: *if you prescribe it, you are liable!* If patient is unconscious, check notes thoroughly (or contact relatives/GP if time). Do not let an incident (or near-incident) be the way you learn this!

PNEUMONIA

1. Community-acquired pneumonia

Severity assessment of community-acquired pneumonia in hospital[1]
Adapted with permission of BMJ group from BTS guidelines.
Thorax 2001; **56** (suppl IV) and 2004 update.
'CURB 65' score – 1 point each for:

Confusion; MTS[2] $\leqslant$ 8/10 **or** *new* disorientation in time, place or person
Urea > 7 mmol/l
Respiratory rate $\geqslant$ 30/min
BP$\downarrow$: systolic < 90 mmHg **or** diastolic $\leqslant$ 60 mmHg
65: age $\geqslant$ 65 yrs

- **<2: Non-severe***; likely suitable for home treatment.
- **2: Severe**** with *increased* risk of death; consider admission (or hospital supervised outpatient care) using clinical judgement.
- **>2: Severe**** with *high* risk of death; admit and consider HDU/ITU (esp if ≥4).

[1] For assessment in the community use '*CRB-65*', which doesn't need blood test: 0 = likely suitable for home treatment; 1–2 = consider hospital referral; 3–4 = urgent hospital admission.
[2] MTS = (Abbreviated) Mental Test Score; see p. 217 for details.

Treatment:

Non-severe**:* amoxicillin 500 mg – 1.0 g tds po
± erythromycin*** 500 mg qds po (if admitted for clinical reasons).
Severe**:* co-amoxiclav 1.2 g tds iv + erythromycin*** 500 mg qds iv.
± flucloxacillin 1 g qds iv if *S. aureus* (Hx or epidemic of 'flu).
± rifampicin 600 mg bd po/iv if *Legionella* (do urinary Ag test).

- If no improvement, change co-amoxiclav to 2nd-generation cephalosporin (e.g. cefuroxime 0.75–1.5 g tds iv).
- If risk factors, consider Rx for aspiration or TB as below.
- If penicillin hypersensitivity, use erythromycin*** only.
- GI intolerance (esp N&V) of erythromycin*** is common; change to clarithromycin 500 mg bd po/iv.

Causes of community-acquired pneumonia (UK adults)
Adapted with permission of BMJ group from Lim, W.S. *et al*. *Thorax* 2001; **56**: 296–301.

48% *Streptococcus pneumoniae:* esp in winter or shelters/prison.
23% **viruses:** influenza (A ≫ B), RSV, rhinoviruses, adenoviruses.
15% *Chlamydia psittaci:* esp from animals, but only 20% from birds (less commonly *Chlamydia pneumoniae*, esp if long-term Hx and headache).
7% *Haemophilus influenzae.*

3% **Mycoplasma pneumoniae:** ↑s during 4-yearly epidemics.
3% **Legionella pneumophila:** ↑d if recent travel (esp Turkey, Spain).
2% **Moraxella catarrhalis:** ↑d in elderly.
1.5% **Staphylococcus aureus:** mostly post-influenza ∴ ↑s in winter.
1.4% **Gram-negative infection:** E. coli, Pseudomonas, Klebsiella,
        Proteus, Serratia.
1.1% **Anaerobes:** e.g. Bacteroides, Fusobacterium.
0.7% **Coxiella burnetii:** ↑s in April–June and in sheep farmers.

NB: 25% are mixed aetiology (accounts for total of >100%).
In ≥20% of cases, causative pathogen is not identified.

The term 'atypical pathogens' is not considered useful by the
BTS (refers to *Mycoplasma, Chlamydia, Coxiella, Legionella*) as
there is no characteristic clinical presentation for the pneumonias
they cause.

2. Hospital-acquired pneumonia

Non-severe: co-amoxiclav 625 mg tds po.
Severe: 3rd-generation cephalosporin, e.g. ceftriaxone 1 g od iv
(max 4 g/day) or cefotaxime 1 g tds iv (max 2 g qds). Ceftazidime
1 g tds iv (max 2 g tds) can be used if complicated infection
(see below), if *Pseudomonas* suspected or if failure to improve.
± metronidazole 500 mg tds iv if aspiration suspected.
± gentamicin if septic shock or failure to improve.
MRSA: teicoplanin/vancomycin if confirmed colonisation/infection.

Causes of hospital-acquired pneumonia
Reproduced with permission from Hammersmith Hospitals NHS
Trust Clinical Management Guidelines & Formulary 2001.

- **Simple:** (w/in 7 days of admission): *H. influenzae, S. pneumoniae,
  S. aureus,* Gram-negative organisms (see top of page).
- **Complicated*:** Gram-negative organisms (esp *P. aeruginosa*),
  Acinebacter, MRSA.
- **Anaerobic*:** *Bacteroides, Fusobacterium.*

- Special situations:
   1 Head trauma, coma, DM, RF: consider *S. aureus*.
   2 Mini-epidemics in hospitals: consider *Legionella*.

*>7 days after admission, recent multiple antibiotics or complex medical Hx (e.g. recent ITU/recurrent admissions or severe comorbidity).

**esp if risk of aspiration, recent abdominal surgery, bronchial obstruction/poor dentition.

3. Aspiration pneumonia

Treatment as for community- or hospital-acquired pneumonia,
+ metronidazole 500 mg tds po/iv.

4. Cavitating pneumonia

Co-amoxiclav 1.2 g tds iv + flucloxacillin 1 g qds iv.
NB: need to exclude TB with sputum/Heaf test ± pleural Bx.

'TANKS' cause cavitation: TB, *Aspergillus*, *Nocardia*, *Klebsiella*,
S. aureus (and *pSeudomonas*).

TB

Get expert advice from respiratory/microbiology departments.
NB: contact consultant in communicable disease control.
Rx normally comes in two phases:

- *Initial phase:* for 1st 2 months: ↓s bacterial load and covers all
   strains: Rifater* (**R**ifampicin + **I**soniazid + **P**yrazinamide) +
   Ethambutol = '**RIPE**'.
- *Continuation phase:* for next 4 months: Rifinah* or Rimactazid*
   (**R**ifampicin + **I**soniazid) = '**RI**'. If resistance to rifampicin/
   isoniazid known (or suspected), continue **P**yrazinamide = '**RIP**'.
- Combined tablets* ⇒ ↑compliance and ease of prescribing.
- All doses are by weight; see BNF for details.
- All are hepatotoxic: check LFTs before and during Rx.
- **Ethambutol** is nephrotoxic and can ⇒ optic neuritis**: check
   U&Es and visual acuity before and during Rx. Alternative is
   streptomycin (also nephrotoxic), but both can be omitted if ↓risk
   of isoniazid resistance.

ACUTE BRONCHITIS

Rx not usually needed in previously healthy patients <60 years old.

- *COPD:* 1st-line: amoxicillin 500 mg tds po/iv.
  2nd-line: co-amoxiclav, erythromycin or doxycycline.
- *Bronchiectasis:* cefuroxime 750 mg tds iv (co-amoxiclav po if mild).
- *Cystic fibrosis:* ciprofloxacin 500 mg bd po (or 400 mg bd ivi) if *Pseudomonas* suspected. Otherwise try gentamicin + piperacillin until sensitivities known.

UPPER RESPIRATORY TRACT AND ENT INFECTIONS

- *Acute epiglottitis:* cefotaxime 1 g tds iv + metronidazole 500 mg tds iv (ceftriaxone alone should suffice in children).
- *Pharyngitis/tonsillitis* (sore/'Strep' throat): penicillin V (phenoxymethylpenicillin) 500 mg tds po if Hx of otitis media, confirmed group A Strep infection or 3 of the following 4 clues that infection is not viral: purulent tonsils, Hx of fever, lack of cough or cervical lymphadenopathy.
- *Sinusitis/otitis media:* amoxicillin 500 mg tds po if local pus or if does not resolve in 2–3 days (as would expect if viral aetiology).
- *Otitis externa:* mostly bacterial; give topical Sofradex or Otomize. Less commonly fungal (look for black spores); give topical Otosporin or Neo-cortef. If does not resolve or evidence of perichondritis (inflamed pinna), cellulitis, boils or local abscess, refer to ENT for specialist advice and consideration of systemic Rx (e.g. amoxicillin, co-amoxiclav, flucloxacillin) and local toilet (esp if fungal).

URINARY TRACT INFECTIONS

- *Simple UTI:* trimethoprim 200 mg bd po. Another option is nitrofurantoin 50–100 mg qds po (not suitable if RF).
- *Pyelonephritis (suspect if loin pain/systemic features):* cefotaxime 1 g tds iv. If no response within 24 h (and still no culture results), try ampicillin 1 g qds iv + gentamicin.

> **Causes of UTIs**
> Mnemonic = '**SEEK** Pee Pee':
> *S. aureus** (*S. saprophyticus*, *S. epidermis* ↑d in women).
> *E. coli*: 70–80% of cases (penicillin resistance common).
> *Enterococci**, e.g. *Streptococcus faecalis*.
> *K*lebsiella**
> *P*roteus mirabilis**
> *P*seudomonas.
> Others: *Candida* (esp if urinary catheter), *Serratia*.
> *↑d if renal stones or recent instrumentation (e.g. cystoscopy).
> **↑d if renal stones, recent instrumentation, obstructive uropathy or recurrent infections.

GI INFECTIONS

Gastroenteritis

- Simple infections rarely need Rx; focus on rehydration and contact microbiology department if in doubt.
- *AAC (*Clostridium difficile*): metronidazole 400 mg tds po and stop other antibiotics if possible.* If no response after 6 days, change to vancomycin 125 mg qds po for 7–10 days.

H. pylori eradication: 'triple therapy'

Give 7-day course (if relapse or maltoma give for 14 days).

1 *Antibiotic 1:* amoxicillin 1 g bd po.
2 + *Antibiotic 2:* clarithromycin 500 mg bd po (or metronidazole 400 mg tds if previous eradication failure).
3 + *Acid suppressant:* PPI (e.g. lansoprazole 30 mg bd) or ranitidine bismuth citrate 400 mg bd (NB: ≠ 'normal' ranitidine!).

Lansoprazole is available in combination packs with amoxicillin + clarithromycin as Heliclear: simpler to prescribe and ↑compliance.

MALARIA

Clues: fevers (±3-day cycles ± rigors), ↓Pt, ↓Hb, jaundice, ↑spleen/liver, travel (even >1 year previously).

Always consult infectious diseases ± microbiology team if malaria suspected/confirmed.

If confirmed non-falciparum ('benign'):

- Chloroquine: initial dose 600 mg po, then 300 mg 6–8 h later, then 300 mg od 24 h later for 2 days (all doses of chloroquine as *base*). Follow, unless pregnant, with primaquine if *P. ovale* or *P. vivax* to kill parasites in the liver and prevent relapses (as a 'radical cure').

If falciparum ('malignant') or species mixed/unknown:
If seriously ill (e.g. ↓GCS), get senior help and give:

- Quinine: load* with 20 mg/kg ivi (max 1.4 g) over 4 h. After 8 h, give 10 mg/kg (max 700 mg) iv over 4 h every 8 h for up to 7 days (↓doses to 5–7 mg/kg if RF or >48 h iv Rx needed), changing to oral quinine (600 mg tds) once able to swallow and retain tablets to complete a 7-day course. Mefloquine is an alternative to oral quinine after 2–3 days of iv quinine (starting ≥12 h after last iv dose).
- Consider artesunate or artemether: get specialist advice.
- Fansidar: 3 tablets as single dose following the course of quinine (each tablet = pyrimethamine 25 mg + sulfadoxine 200 mg) if quinine resistance know or suspected. Doxycycline 200 mg od po for ≥7 days is used instead if Fansidar resistance.

If stable, normal GCS, and able to swallow and retain tablets:

- Quinine: 600 mg tds po for 7 days followed by doxycycline, clindamycin or Fansidar if quinine resistance known or suspected. Proguanil + atovaquone (Malarone), artemether + lumefantrine (Riamet) or mefloquine are alternatives to quinine and don't need any subsequent drugs.

☙Quinine doses here are as **salt** (specify this on prescription): don't confuse with **base**, which has different doses. *Don't give iv loading dose if quinine, quinidine or mefloquine given in past 24h.

MENINGITIS

Empirical Rx (until results of LP known – esp Gram stain).

- Cefotaxime 2 g qds ivi: Rx of choice for *N. meningitides* (aka meningococcus; commonest cause in UK adults). If Hx of hypersensitivity to cephalosporins (or penicillins as 10% also hypersensitive to cephalosporins) consider chloramphenicol iv instead.

Consider:

- Ampicillin 2 g 4 hourly iv + gentamicin iv if *Listeria* suspected, e.g. immunosuppression or indicative CSF: non-TB Gram-positive bacilli.
- Aciclovir 10 mg/kg over 1 h tds iv if HSV encephalitis suspected, e.g. more prominent confusion, behavioural Δs and seizures.
- TB Rx as for pneumonia: if risk factors or suggestive CSF findings (↑LØ, ↑protein, ↓glucose).

Causes of meningitis in the UK
Common:
- *N. meningitidis*, serotype B: majority (70–80%) of cases.
- *N. meningitidis*, serotype C: ↓ing secondary to vaccine.
- *N. meningitidis*, serotype A: ↑ing again (had been ↓ing).
- *S. pneumoniae*: stable incidence.

Rarer:
- Gram-negative bacilli.
  Listeria monocytogenes: esp neonates, age >60, ↓immunity.
- *H. influenzae*, type b: ↓ing secondary to vaccine.

Don't forget:
- Viral: HSV/HZV, EBV, HIV, mumps: esp if encephalitic (↓GCS).
  Less commonly entero/echo/coxsackie/polio viruses.
- TB, other bacteria, e.g. *Borrelia*: esp if ↓immunity/HIV.
- Fungi: cryptococcus, candida: esp if ↓immunity/HIV.
- Group B *Streptococcus*: predominantly in neonates.
- *S. aureus*: if neurosurgery, ↓immunity, invasive lines, IVDU.

EYE INFECTIONS

For conjunctivitis, blepharitis* and corneal abrasions:

- chloramphenicol 0.5% 1 drop 2 hrly reducing to qds + 0.5% ointment to lids od nocte.
  ± doxycycline po if systemic Rx required* (not for children).
  Consult ophthalmologist for advice if at all unsure (extra care needed if contact lens wearer).

CELLULITIS

Mild (e.g. Venflon site infection): co-amoxiclav 375 mg tds po.
Severe: benzylpenicillin 1.2 g 4–6 hourly + flucloxacillin 1 g qds iv.
+ metronidazole 500 mg tds iv if suspect anaerobes, e.g. abdominal wound.
+ consider vancomycin if confirmed MRSA colonisation/infection.

BONE AND JOINT INFECTIONS

Osteomyelitis: suspect in any postoperative joint or deep DM ulcer.

- Flucloxacillin 1 g qds iv + fusidic acid 1 g tds po (can give iv in severe cases, but is poorly tolerated and often not required; see main drugs section for doses).

Septic arthritis: suspect if sudden-onset pain/inflammation.

- Treatment as osteomyelitis, but consider changing after urgent Gram stain, e.g. to iv 3rd-generation cephalosporin (e.g. cefotaxime, ceftriaxone) if *H. influenzae* suspected (Gram-negative bacilli, esp in children). Suspect *Salmonella* in sickle cell disease or TB/fungi if immunocompromised.

PUO

No routine antibiotics indicated, but suspect and exclude abdominal abscess, TB, Ca (esp abdominal/haematological) and other causes.

Causes of PUO

- Faulty thermometer/poor technique (e.g. oral temp after hot drink!).
- Abdominal abscess: liver, subphrenic, pelvic.
- Other infection: UTI, TB, malaria, SBE, virus (EBV, CMV, HIV).
- Autoimmune: rheumatoid arthritis, Still's disease, PMR, sarcoid, PAN, SLE/connective tissue disease.
- Cancer: lymphoma, leukaemia, solid tumours (esp abdominal).
- Drugs: almost any (inc drugs of abuse), often assoc w ↑EØ.
- Other: PEs, haematomas, alcoholic hepatitis, FMF.

NB: up to 25% of cases remain unexplained.

NEUTROPENIA

If temperature 38°C for ⩾2 h (or ⩾38.5°C for ⩾1 h) and no clues as to the fever's aetiology, give:

- *For 1st/2nd episodes:* gentamicin 5 mg/kg od iv + Tazocin 4.5 g tds iv (use ceftazidime 2 g tds iv if penicillin allergy).
- *For persistent or recurrent fever at any later stage:* call haematologist/oncologist ± microbiologist on call for advice.

NB: always do full septic screen before giving/prescribing antibiotics: blood, urine and any other appropriate cultures (e.g. sputum, stool, central/other lines) ± CXR.

HYPERTENSION MANAGEMENT

Adapted with permission of BMJ group from Joint British Societies (includes BHS) guidelines. *Heart* 2005 **91** (suppl 5): 1–52.

When to treat: depends on severity and other factors:

Severity	Systolic[1]	OR	Diastolic[1]	Drug therapy[2]
Normal	<120		<80	No
High-normal	135–139		85–89	Consider[3]
Mild (Grade 1)	140–159		90–99	Consider[4]

Severity	Systolic[1]	OR	Diastolic[1]	Drug therapy[2]
Moderate (Grade 2)	160–179		100–109	Yes
Severe (Grade 3)	≥180		≥110	Yes

1. All measurements are in mmHg. 2. Encourage lifestyle modifications *for all* ↑BP: ↓salt, ↓Wt, ↓alcohol, stop smoking, ↑exercise, ↑fresh fruit/vegetables, ↓intake of total and unsaturated fat. For mild and high-normal cases without CVD or target organ damage* these measures can be tried before drug therapy. 3. May be indicated if established CVD, chronic renal disease, or DM with complications at BP levels >130/80 mmHg. 4. Recommended if established CVD or DM, or evidence of target organ damage*, or 10-yr CVD risk ≥20% (see risk charts at back of BNF or at www.bhsoc.org/resources/prediction chart.htm).

*HF, established IHD, CVA/TIA, abnormal renal function (↑creatinine or proteinuria/micoalbuminuria), hypertensive/diabetic retinopathy or LVH.

☠ *See p. 199 for Dx and Mx of accelerated HTN.* ☠

Aim for: BP ≤140/85 mmHg. If DM or CRF ≤130/80 mmHg. If CRF and >1 g/24 h proteinuria ≤120/75.

Primary causes: look for and exclude (esp if treatable), e.g. RAS, Conn's (1° hyperaldosteronism), ↑Ca^{2+}, Cushing's, phaeo (esp if variable BP, headaches, sweats, palpitations) and recreational drugs (e.g. alcohol, cocaine, amphetamines).

NB: stress (inc 'white-coat HTN'), recreational drug use and withdrawal (esp alcohol) are common temporary causes.

Important points:

- Make a *written* Rx plan for (other) doctors, nurses and patient. Include target BP and how Rx should change if it is not achieved.
- Age/ethnic origin influence response to drugs (see table below).
- A single agent is rarely successful at achieving target BP. Rather than ↑ing doses, add 2nd and 3rd agents, which often work in an additive or complementary fashion, esp if table below used.
- Exclude/minimise NSAID use, inc unrecognized 'over-the-counter' use, as reason for poor treatment response.

Choice of Drug: Rational Combination Therapy ('Cambridge AB/CD Rule')

Step	Younger (< 55 years) and non-black	Older (≥ 55 years) or black[1]
1	A (or B[2])	C or D
2	A (or B[3]) + C or D	
3	A (or B[3]) + C + D	
4	Resistant hypertension[4]	

1. Black = African (not Asian) origin. 2. B is less preferred as less effective but consider if angina, post-MI or chronic stable LVF. 3. B is less preferred as could mean combination of two diabetogenic drugs (e.g. β-blocker + diuretic), esp in elderly. 4. Add α-blocker, spironolactone or other diuretic ⇒ specialist referral and consider missed 1° cause or poor compliance.

☺ good for, ☹ avoid/caution, ☠ beware!

A = ACE-i, e.g. enalapril initially 5 mg od (2.5 mg if elderly or RF). ☺ CRF (but *with caution!*), HF, DM, IHD. ☹ PVD (as assoc with RAS*). ☠ Pregnancy, bilateral RAS*. (*Must check U&Es 2 wks after starting, esp if vasculopathy or renal impairment*).
    Angiotensin II receptor blockers (ARBs) can also be used but are normally reserved for when ACE-i not tolerated (esp dt dry cough).
B = β-blocker, e.g. atenolol 50 mg od. ☺ anxiety, IHD (post-MI/angina), chronic stable LVF. ☹ dyslipidaemia, PVD, DM (unless also IHD), if on diltiazem. ☠ asthma/COPD, HB, acute LVF, if on verapamil.
C = Ca²⁺-channel blocker: dihydropyridines such as amlodipine 5 mg or nifedipine LA (e.g. **Adalat LA** 20–30 mg od) usually 1st-line. ☺ elderly. ☹ oedema. ☠ aortic stenosis, recent ACS.
If IHD 'rate-limiting' types (verapamil, diltiazem) often preferred. ☠ HF, HB, if on other rate-limiting drugs (esp β-blockers).
D = diuretic, e.g. bendroflumethiazide 2.5 mg od. ☺ oedema/HF, elderly, isolated systolic HTN, 2°CVA prevention. ☹ dyslipidaemia. ☠ gout.

NB: only starting doses are given; see main drugs section or SPCs/BNF for doses thereafter.

When to change Rx (after checking compliance first!):
- BP < 5 mmHg lower: if HTN mild and uncomplicated, switch across 'AB' or 'CD' category of drug, i.e. from A (or B) *to* C or D

(or vice versa). If HTN severe or complicated, add 2nd agent as per table above.

- BP > 5 mmHg lower but:
  - drug not tolerated: swap within category, i.e. from A* *to* B (or vice versa) or from C *to* D (or vice versa);
  - still suboptimal: either ↑dose or add 2nd agent (often better).

Consider swapping from ACE-i to ARB (or vice versa) as β-blockers often less preferable, as above.

ASTHMA

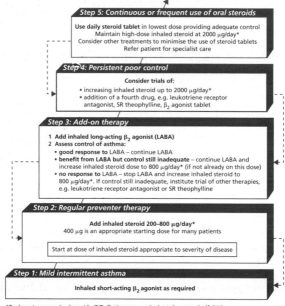

*Beclometasone or budesonide (NB: fluticasone equivalent doses are half this).

Figure 1 BTS guidelines for management of asthma in adults. Adapted with permission of BMJ group from *Thorax* 2003; **58** (suppl 1): 24.

PEF PREDICTOR FOR 'WRIGHTS' (OLD SCALE) MEASUREMENTS

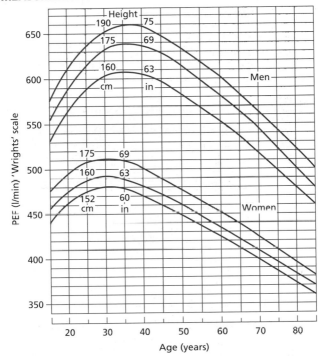

Figure 2 Peak expiratory flow (PEF) predictor for normal adults using 'Wrights' (Wright–McKerrow) scale. Check PEF meter used was not calibrated to the new 'EU' scale, which is replacing the 'Wrights' scale; if so use Figure 3.
Adapted with permission of BMJ group from Gregg, I. and Nunn, A.J. *British Medical Journal* 1989; **298**: 1098.

PEF PREDICTOR FOR 'EU' (NEW SCALE) MEASUREMENTS

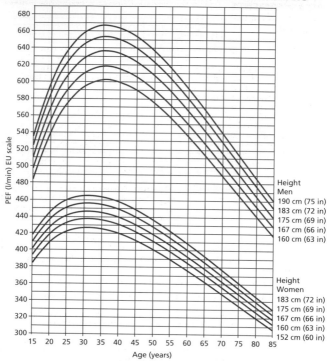

Figure 3 Peak expiratory flow (PEF) predictor for normal adults using new European standard 'EU' (EN 13826) scale. Check the PEF meter used was not calibrated to the old 'Wrights' scale which is being phased out; if so use Figure 2. Adapted with permission of BMJ group from Gregg, I. and Nunn, A.J. *British Medical Journal* 1989; **298**: 1098, corrected to the EN 13826: 2003 scale values by Clement Clarke International Ltd.

ANALGESIA

Choice of analgesic:

General rules
- Look for/treat reversible causes and reassess cause at each step.
- Regular Rx ↓s relapses *but always review to check whether still needed.*
- If pain ↓s, 'step down' and ensure adequate pm analgesia in case ↑s again.
- Pain has many adverse medical fx and is rarely refractory to the correct Rx.
- If pain persists, get senior or specialist help (e.g. anaesthetist or pain team).

- All opioids can ⇒ constipation,
  respiratory depression and ↓GCS
  (esp if elderly or RF – even low
  doses). Can also ⇒ coma if LF.
- All NSAIDs can ⇒ PU; related to
  strength of drug and length
  of Rx. Consider PPI or changing
  to COX2 inhibitor[NICE].

Step 4
- Strong opioid:
  iv if acute (e.g. morphine)
  po if chronic (e.g. oramorph)
  ± sc pump: see p. 156

Step 3
- High dose mild opioid e.g.:
  – codeine phosphate 30–60 mg qds
  – tramadol 50–100 mg qds (also has
    5HT fx: ↓SEs for same analgesia)

Step 2
- Compound prep. of paracetamol with low dose mild
  opioid (e.g. cocodamol or codydramol)
- Stronger NSAID: e.g. naproxen, keterolac or indometacin

Step 1
- **Simple analgesia:** paracetamol 1 g qds usually 1st-line as few SEs.

  NSAIDs usually 2nd-line unless predominant inflammatory component, e.g.:
  – Ibuprofen 200–400 mg tds po for mild pain.
  – Diclofenac (Voltarol) 50 mg tds im/po or 75 mg bd im/po or 100 mg pr
    (max 150 mg/day) for moderate pain (esp good postoperatively).

- **Consider specialist analgesia** according to cause, e.g. buscopan for colic,
  colchicine for gout, antacids for reflux, GTN for angina. For neuropathic
  pain try amitriptyline, gabapentin or pregabalin.

Figure 4 Analgesia ladder. Based on WHO pain relief ladder for cancer pain.

NB: it is often worth persevering with simple analgesia even when strong opiates are used as
they have additive fx in combination (esp in combination with paracetamol).

Important points for postoperative patients:

- Oral route often ineffective *for all operations* (due to gastric
  stasis).

- Epidural anaesthesia (EDA) and patient-controlled analgesia (PCA) normally provide maximal opiates (as well as other drugs) ∴ beware of giving more. Try strong NSAID as below and get advice from anaesthetist if this does not work.
- Consider local/regional anaesthesia.

PALLIATIVE CARE AND SUBCUTANEOUS PUMPS

- Underprescribed due to stigma of being a 'final measure': ensure good communication with patient, relatives and nurses as to reasons for use.
- Gives smooth symptom control, esp for pain, but also useful for other symptoms, e.g. nausea, xs secretions, agitation. Good if unable to take po medications, avoids cannulation, only single 24-h prescription needed (no delays in drug administration on busy wards).
- Palliative care, Macmillan and hospital pain teams will help if unsure of the indications or how to set up these pumps.

CONTENTS

1 *Diamorphine:* calculate dose needed for 24-h prescription from the past 24 hours' requirements (if variable, look at longer-term trend). If taking other opioids, use the following *rough* guide:

$$1 \, mg \, diamorphine \, sc = 3 \, mg \, morphine \, po$$
$$= 15 \, mg \, tramadol \, po$$
$$= 25 \, mg \, pethidine \, im$$
$$= 35 \, mg \, codeine \, po/im$$

(For conversion from fentanyl, see its entry in main drugs section.)

NB: this table applies only for the specific route(s) of each drug stated, as bioavailability can vary widely with routes. Also, it does not take into account duration of action, although this can be ignored if 24-h requirements for each drug are calculated.

2 Antiemetic: choose from (*generally start at lowest dose*):
   - Metoclopramide 30–100 mg/24 h: normally 1st choice
     (esp for promotility fx to counter opioid constipation; but CI
     if GI obstruction!).
   - Haloperidol 2.5–5 mg/24h: good general antiemetic.
   - Levomepromazine 6.25–12.5 mg/24 h. Good if cause unknown
     or multifactorial (↑doses to 25–50 mg/h if sedation needed).

3 *Optional extras:*
   - Drugs to ↓respiratory secretions:
     – glycopyrronium 0.6–1.2 mg/24 h: becoming more popular.
     – hyoscine hydrobromide 0.6–2.4 mg/24h: normally sedative
       but can ⇒ paradoxical agitation.
   - Sedatives, e.g. midazolam 20–100 mg/24h if restlessness
     or agitation is the solitary symptom or refractory to
     levomepromazine. Care/↓dose if elderly, respiratory
     depression, benzodiazepine-naïve.

Compatibility of drugs in syringe drivers

It is advised that only two or three drugs are used per syringe
driver. All antiemetics listed above are compatible with
diamorphine. For addition of 'optional extras', see table below;
for all other combinations, check with the hospital pharmacy or
drug information office. Out-of-hours authoritative information
on compatibility (and other palliative care prescribing issues) can
be found at the excellent website www.palliativedrugs.com.

Compatibility* of specific three-drug combinations: diamorphine and antiemetic
and one other 'optional extra' drug.

Diamorphine *plus*	Glycopyrronium	Hyoscine *hydrobromide*	Midazolam
Metoclopramide	Not recommended	Not recommended	Compatible*
Haloperidol	Not known	Compatible*	Compatible*
Levomepromazine	Compatible*	Compatible*	Compatible*

*Compatibility is restricted to usual dose ranges of the drugs.

EXAMPLE PRESCRIPTION

Prescribe each drug individually in the 'regular prescriptions' section
of the drug chart, as shown here:

DATE/ TIME	INFUSION FLUID	VOL- UME	ADDITIVES IF ANY DRUG AND DOSE	RATE OF ADMIN	DURA- TION	DR'S SIGNATURE	TIME START- ED	TIME COMP- LETED	SET UP BY SIG- NATURE	BATCH No.
08/01	Water for injection	48 ml	+ Diamorphine 60 mg			TH				
			+ Metoclopramide 30 mg							
	Total of 48 ml to run subcutaneously via syringe driver at 2 ml per hour over 24 h									

Figure 5 Example drug chart of diamorphine subcutaneous pump. *NB: 60 mg diamorphine/24 h is **example dose**; individual patient needs will vary (see p. 156).*

> *Graseby syringe drivers: **mm** (instead of **ml**) per unit time*
> This type of syringe driver is common in the UK (esp in specialist palliative care settings). Infusions are given in **millimetres (mm)** rather than **millilitres (ml)** per unit time. There are 2 types: for each unit on the 'rate' dial, the MS16 (blue) delivers 1 mm/**h**, but the MS26 (green) delivers 1 mm/**day**. The prescription in Figure 5 (in ml) is still valid but will need to be translated into mm by the person setting up driver, so it is simplest to prescribe in mm as follows.
>
> Examples of prescriptions of a syringe to be given over 24 h:
> - **MS16:** 'Diamorphine 60 mg over 24 h as subcutaneous infusion via syringe driver. Mix with water for injection to a length of 48 mm in syringe, set at rate of 2 mm/h.'
> - **MS26:** 'Diamorphine 60 mg over 24 h as subcutaneous infusion via syringe driver. Mix with water for injection to a length of 48 mm in syringe, set at rate of 48 mm/24 h.'
>
> ☠ **Confusing mm with ml or confusing the 2 types of driver can lead to significant differences in rate of drug delivery.** ☠

GENERAL POINTERS IN CHRONIC PAIN/ PALLIATIVE CARE

- *Laxatives:* give with opiates as Px rather than later as Rx.
- *Fentanyl patches:* smooth pain control w/o multiple injections or tablets (just change patch every 3rd day). Also less constipating.
- *Breakthrough analgesia:* always write up in case regular medications become insufficient. Oral opiates (e.g. Oramorph) often best; 1/6th of regular 24-h opiate equivalent dose is usually sufficient. If ↓GCS or ↓swallow add sc or iv drugs (e.g. morphine).

- *Simple analgesia:* do not forget as often effective, e.g. paracetamol.
- *Steroids:* consider for nausea, as pain adjuvant (esp liver capsule pain), and for short-term Rx of ↓appetite: get specialist help.
- *Always consider new causes of pain/distress*, esp if patient unable to give Hx: often treatable, iatrogenic or can be disguised/made worse by more analgesia, e.g. opiate-induced constipation, patient positioning, UTI, urinary retention, mental anguish (esp 'unfinished business'), pathological fractures.

Commonly missed problems

- ↑Ca^{2+}: esp consider if confusion and constipation (other symptoms: 'bones, stones, groans and psychic moans'); see pp. 209–10 for Mx.
- *Spinal cord compression:* ↑back pain, sensory/sphincter disturbance, limb weakness – *can be treated* with immediate high-dose steroids (e.g. dexamethasone phosphate 12–16 mg iv then 8 mg po bd) and radiotherapy.

ANTIEMETICS

General rules

- Look for/treat reversible causes (see below).
- Reassess causes at each step.
- Start iv/im (and switch to po ASAP).
- Consider sc pump if chronic (see p. 156).
- Don't stop Rx unless cause removed.

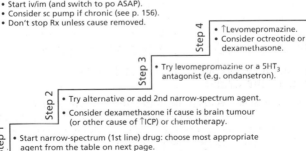

Step 4
- ↑Levomepromazine.
- Consider octreotide or dexamethasone.

Step 3
- Try levomepromazine or a $5HT_3$ antagonist (e.g. ondansetron).

Step 2
- Try alternative or add 2nd narrow-spectrum agent.
- Consider dexamethasone if cause is brain tumour (or other cause of ↑ICP) or chemotherapy.

Step 1
- Start narrow-spectrum (1st line) drug: choose most appropriate agent from the table on next page.

Figure 6 Antiemetic ladder – designed for cancer patients; steps 3 and 4 rarely needed in other settings.

Commonly used 1st line/narrow-spectrum antiemetics (see also Palliative care section, pp. 156–9).

Class	Example	Good for	Beware
Phenothiazine (D_2 antagonist)	**Prochlorperazine** 10–20 mg po or 12.5 mg im (Stemetil)	Opiates, general anaesthetic, postoperative, chemo-/radio-therapy (if mild)	⇒ ↑prolactin, extrapyramidal fx, ↓s seizure threshold, ↓BP
Benzamine (D_2 antagonist)	**Metoclopramide** 10 mg tds po/im/iv (Maxolon)	GI causes (↑s GI motility*), migraine, drugs (esp opiates)	⇒ ↑prolactin, extrapyramidal fx, ⊗ CI if GI obstruction * ⊗
Benzamine (D_2 antagonist)	**Domperidone** 10–20 mg tds po or 30–60 mg tds pr (not iv or im)	Parkinson's disease**, morning-after pill, chemotherapy	⇒ ↑prolactin, but minimal sedation and extrapyramidal fx**
Antihistamines	**Cyclizine** 50 mg tds po/im/iv	GI obstruction*/postoperative N&V, vestibular/labyrinthine disorders	⇒ Antimuscarinic fx (esp sedation). Avoid in IHD (↓s beneficial cardiodynamic fx of opiates)
5HT$_3$ antagonists	**Ondansetron** 8 mg bd po/im/iv (16 mg od pr) **Granisetron** **Tropisetron**	Severe/resistant cases (esp chemotherapy)	Minimal side effects: headache, constipation, dizziness

Causes of nausea
- *Drugs:* esp opiates, chemotherapy/cytotoxics. Commonly also dopamine agonists, antibiotics (esp erythromycin), antidepressants (esp fluoxetine), theophyllines, colchicine, $FeSO_4$ and acutely amiodarone/digoxin.
- *GI:* constipation, but also surgical (obstruction, peritonism) and medical (oesophagitis, gastritis, PU) causes.
- *Neurological:* migraine, $\uparrow$ICP (esp tumour), meningitis, Menière's, labyrinthitis.
- *Metabolism:* $\uparrow Ca^{2+}$ (also $\downarrow Na^+$, $\uparrow K^+$), DM, ARF, Addison's.
- *Infection:* gastroenteritis but also UTI, respiratory infections.
- *Other:* pregnancy, MI (esp inferior, often $\downarrow$pain if DM/elderly).

ALCOHOL WITHDRAWAL

A 'detox' programme comprises the following components:

1. PREVENTION OF AGITATION, SEIZURES AND DELIRIUM TREMENS

Give a long-acting benzodiazepine in a tapered regimen as follows:

Alcohol withdrawal regimen. With permission from Professor H. Ghodse, St George's Hospital.

Day	Chlordiazepoxide	OR	Diazepam
1	30 mg qds		15 mg qds
2	30 mg tds		10 mg qds
3	20 mg tds		10 mg tds
4	20 mg bd		5 mg qds
5	10 mg bd		5 mg tds
6	10 mg od		5 mg bd
7	10 mg prn		5 mg od

These are only suggested initial average regimens. Requirements vary considerably with severity of symptoms and previous experience of or tolerance to benzodiazepines. Regular dose review and prescription of prn doses is essential. Ideal regimens involve an initial 24-h assessment of prn doses, but require

162) DRUG SELECTION

adequate training and time of staff to monitor closely and ensure no under- (or over-) treatment occurs. Start with dose of 20–40 mg chlordiazepoxide or 10–20 mg diazepam and add up doses used in 1st 24 h, then reduce by 1/5th (–1/7th) per day for 5(–7) days.

- Chlordiazepoxide usually first line, but diazepam preferred if Hx of seizures (esp if occurred in context of alcohol withdrawal).
- If significant liver failure (e.g. ↑AST or ALT), consider shorter acting benzodiazepines such as oxazepam or lorazepam at equivalent doses (see p. 190); avoids xs metabolite build up and sedation.
- Only start once acute alcohol intoxication has resolved as benzodiazepines are contraindicated in this state.

2. THIAMINE (VIT B1) AND OTHER SUPPLEMENTS

For Px or Rx of Wernicke's encephalopathy (WE): must give before patient receives carbohydrate load po or iv, which can precipitate WE.

☠ ∴ Take particular care if hypoglycaemic and iv glucose needed! ☠

- **Parenteral (iv or im) thiamine:** e.g. Pabrinex (contains other B and C vits); prescribe as '1 pair pabrinex vials' or 'Pabrinex 1 and 2'. British Association of Psychopharmacology guidelines 2004 recommend:
  - If WE established (or *suspected*; see note box below): 2 pairs tds iv (or im) for 3 days, then 1 pair od for 3–5 days.
  - If high risk of WE (malnourished/chronic severe abuse): 1 pair od iv im for 3–5 days.
  - If low risk of WE no parenteral treatment needed.

☠ Pabrinex **can** ⇒ **anaphylaxis** ∴ ensure resus facilities at hand. NB: ↑risk if given iv too quickly; ensure mixture of both vials either given as injection over ≥ 10 min or as infusion (with 50–100 ml saline) over ≥30 min. ☠

- Oral vitamins and supplements.
  - Thiamine 100 mg bd/tds po; should be given for 1 month if no parenteral treatment required.
  - Multivitamins 1 tablet/day long-term; cheap and potentially important if future diet unlikely to be good.

Wernicke's encephalopathy (WE)
Caused by thiamine deficiency and often missed; only 10% have classical triad of confusion, ataxia and eye signs (ophthalmoplegia or nystagmus; seen in only 30% of cases). Suspect diagnosis if *any* evidence of chronic alcohol misuse and *any* one of: acute confusion, ataxia, ophthalmoplegia, ↓BP + ↓temp, ↓GCS or ↓memory. If unsure whether intoxication or WE causing any of these, always assume it is WE and give treatment. Rarely WE is caused by other malnutrition, e.g. malabsorption, eating disorders, protracted vomiting, CRF, AIDS and other drug misuse.

---

3. MAINTENANCE OF ABSTINENCE

It is essential to:

- Encourage abstinence and consider referral to addiction services.
- Treat depression and try to arrange adequate social support.

Consider the following as aids:

- *Acamprosate:* ↓s pleasurable fx of alcohol, cravings and relapses.
- *Disulfiram:* ⇒ unpleasant symptoms if alcohol consumed.
- *Naltrexone:* ↓s craving and relapse rate. Specialist use only (not yet licensed in UK for this indication).

How to prescribe

INSULIN

TYPES

Many exist, with differences in the timing of action onset (O), peak (P) and duration (D).

For acute use, e.g. DKA and sliding scales, inc perioperative:

- Soluble (aka normal/neutral) can be given **iv** (and **sc** as other types), e.g. Actrapid, Humulin S:

  iv: O/P immediate, D 0.5 h. **sc:** O 0.5–1 h, P 2–4 h, D 8 h.

For maintenance use, i.e. normal chronic control (sc only):

- **Aspart (▼ NovoRapid), lispro** (Humalog): recombinant human analogues. Rapid onset ⇒ ↑eating flexibility (can give immediately before meals; other types of sc insulin must be given 30 min before), ↓duration ⇒ fewer hypos (esp before meals). O 0.25 h, P 1–3 h, D 2–5 h.
- **Isophane:** Now rarely used in the UK.
- **▼Glargine:** new, long-acting recombinant insulin with delayed and prolonged absorption from sc injection site ⇒ constant, more 'physiological' basal supply; can give od in evening (e.g. Lantus).
- **▼Determir:** new, long-acting analogue. Binds to albumin and has different action from that of glargine but similar advantages. Give od or bd (e.g. Levemir).

SLIDING SCALES

For optimal blood glucose control in diabetics if (i) DKA/HONK, (ii) preoperative/NBM, (iii) MI*/ACS*, (iv) severe concurrent illness (e.g. sepsis).

For MI*/ACS*, ivi of glucose + insulin + K⁺ often preferred (aka GIK or DIGAMI). Use local protocols if they exist; can often be found in CCU or A&E.

Example of how to write an insulin sliding scale on a drug chart

DATE/ TIME	INFUSION FLUID	VOL- UME	ADDITIVES IF ANY DRUG AND DOSE	RATE OF ADMIN	DURA- TION	DR'S SIGNATURE	TIME START- ED	TIME COM- PLETED	SET UP BY SIG- NATURE	BATCH No.
08/01	Normal saline	50 ml	Actrapid 50 units	As below		TN				
08/01	Glucose saline	1 litre								
		CBG (= BM)	INSULIN ivi (ml/h)							
		0–4	0.5 (+ call Dr if CBG < 2.5)							
		4.1–7	1							
		7.1–9	2							
		9.1–11	3							
		11.1–13	4							
		≥ 13.1	6							
Always run glucose saline (4% glucose + 0.18% saline) ivi at 125 ml per hour if CBG (BM) < 15.										

Figure 7 Drug chart, showing slide scale.

These are average requirements and ∴ only a suggested *initial* regimen: requirements will vary widely between individuals and within an individual over time (esp with intercurrent illness, e.g. infections). Regular review and adjustment is essential – see pp. 168–9. Use your hospital's protocols where possible.

Important points

- Check Venflon is working before adjusting sliding scale (may be reason why BG not falling).

- prn insulin (e.g. 2–5 units actrapid sc) can be used when estimated requirements not sufficient. NB: ☠ risk of hypoglycaemia. ☠ Use only when review not possible and if experienced nurses available. Risk can be ↓d by writing on chart that duty doctor must be called to instruct on exact dose to be given. Beware of patients with unpredictable responses to insulin and if patient not known to you.

- Always give glucose* saline (4% glucose and 0.18% saline) ivi at 125 ml/h when CBG <15. If RF or mild HF give 5% glucose* ivi at a slower rate. If severe HF give 10% glucose* (preferably via central line) at 60–70 ml/h. KCl should be added according to individual needs (see pp. 183–4). Write up 50% glucose iv prn in case of severe hypoglycaemia.

- State clearly to nursing staff the frequency with which CBGs are required: very sick patients (e.g. DKA/HONK) need CBGs every half-hour and ideally regular laboratory glucose readings (more accurate). If not very sick and CBGs stable (e.g. preoperative), 2–4-hourly usually suffices.

- Stop oral hypoglycaemics and adjust for residual effects they may be having. Remember to reintroduce before stopping sliding scale!

*NB: glucose = dextrose. Low-strength glucose solutions used to be called dextrose solutions; this is now being phased out.

Amount of insulin: initial doses and adjustment

Prescribe 50 units of soluble insulin (Actrapid or Humulin S) in 50 ml normal saline to run via a syringe driver according to one of the regimens (A, B, C, D) below:

1 Start with regimen A, unless severe insulin resistance (i.e. normally takes ≥100 units sc insulin/day), in which case start with B.

2 If BG >10 (or >7 during acute MI, where target BG even lower) for 3 consecutive hourly tests and is ↑ing (or ↓ing by <25% in

the past hour), step up to next sliding scale (i.e. if on A, step up to B; if on B, step up to C, etc.).

3 If BG <3.5 mmol/l, step down to next scale (i.e. if on B, step down to A; if on C, step down to B, etc.).

Table showing suggested insulin ivi regimens

CBG (= BM)	Insulin ivi (units/h)			
	Regime A	Regime B	Regime C**	Regime D**
0.0–4.0*	0.5	0.5	0.5	0.5
4.1–7.0	1	2	3	4
7.1–9.0	2	4	6	8
9.1–11.0	3	6	9	12
11.1–13.0	4	8	12	16
>13.0	6	12	18	24

*Stop ivi for 15 min if severe hypoglycaemia (CBG <2.5 or symptoms) and give Rx as on p. 206. Otherwise treat more gently with 5–10% glucose ivi and maintain insulin infusion (esp it DKA).
**Rarely needed; used mostly for patients with severe insulin resistance (i.e. on more than 100 units insulin/day before admission).
Reproduced with permission from Prof. S. Kumar, Dr. A. Rahim and Dr. P. Dyer, Endocrinology Department, University of Warwick Medical School.

Coming off a sliding scale
Consider once eating/drinking normally and CBGs normal/stable:

- If post-DKA, change back only if urine free of ketones (ideally, blood ketones should also be checked) and pH back to normal.
- If postoperative and no reason to suppose change in needs (i.e. no infection), go straight back to preoperative regimen.
- Avoid hypos by continuing ivi until 1st sc dose starts to work (usually 10–30 min). Always change from iv to sc before a meal.

The following is only a guide to how to start sc regimens (always consult your hospital's diabetes team if unsure):

1 Calculate daily requirements by doubling the number of units used in the past 12 h from the sliding scale.

2 Start qds sc regimen. If patient is well and CBGs very stable, this step may be omitted (i.e. go straight to a bd regimen). Give 1/3rd of total daily dose at 10pm (as intermediate insulin e.g. Humulin I (i) or Insulatard), then give the rest (as short-acting insulin e.g.

Actrapid or Humulin S) divided equally between
pre-breakfast, pre-lunch and pre-evening meal doses.

3 Start bd sc regimen: give 60% of daily dose pre-breakfast and
   the remaining 40% pre-evening meal, both doses as biphasic
   30/70 insulin (e.g. Humulin M3 or Mixtard 30).

PREOPERATIVE GUIDELINES: GENERAL POINTS (FOR ALL PATIENTS)

Local protocols should be used if they exist, otherwise a sensible
way to progress would be to:

- Ensure patient 1st on operating list and fast from midnight*.
- Stop all long-acting insulins the night before the operation.
- Withhold all DM medications for morning of operation.
- Prescribe 5 or 10% glucose ivi in case of hypoglycaemia.
- Proceed as per table below:

*If pm-only list, give light breakfast and normal morning medications
(but no intermediate/long acting insulins), monitor CBG 1–2-hourly.
Start sliding scale/GIK at 11am (unless well controlled type II) or if
CBGs uncontrolled.

Type of surgery	Type II (control good)		Type II (control poor/ fasting glucose >10) or Type I
		Monitor CBGs 2-hourly	Monitor CBGs 1-hourly
Minor: expect to eat normally the same day	After operation give normal medications ASAP with a meal (sliding scale not usually required).		Start sliding scale/GIK at 10pm the night before op. Give normal medications and meal ASAP after op.
Major/GI: not expected to eat the same day	Start sliding scale/GIK if CBGs not controlled**. Convert back to normal medications once CBGs stable and eating/drinking normally.		Start sliding scale/GIK at 10pm the night before op. Convert back to normal medications once CBGs stable and eating/drinking normally.

**Uncontrolled CBGs = single reading >15 or consistently >10.

ANTICOAGULANTS

WARFARIN

> Consult your hospital anticoagulant service if ever unsure about indications, doses or interactions. Refer as early before discharge as practicable so outpatient monitoring is arranged in time.

Basics

Oral anticoagulant for long-term Rx/Px of TE: loading (see below) usually takes several days, so heparin (quicker-acting) is used as short-term cover until therapeutic levels are achieved.

Monitoring

Via INR = patient's PT (prothrombin time) compared to that of a control. A target INR is set at the start of Rx, according to indication (see below); variations of ±0.5 are acceptable.

BCSH guidelines for target INRs. Adapted with permission from *British Journal of Haematology* 1998; **101**: 374–87 including BCSH 2005 updates.

Indication	Target INR
DVT/PE[1]	2.5
Thrombophilia (if symptomatic)[2]	2.5
Paroxysmal nocturnal haemoglobinuria (PNH)[3]	2.5
AF[4] (or other causes of cardiac emboli[5])	2.5
Bioprosthetic heart valves[6]	2.5
Mechanical heart valves	3.5

1 Treat for ≥6 weeks if calf vein thrombosis, for ≥3 months if proximal DVT/PE, for ≥6 months if ideopathic venous TE or permanent risk factors. If recurrent DVT/PE *whilst on therapeutic Rx*, target INR = 3.5.
2 Arterial thrombosis in antiphospholipid syndrome is exception with target INR 3.5.
3 Treat if large PNH clones (PNH granulocytes >50%) and Pt >100 × 10^9/l. Consider if smaller clones and Pt <100 × 10^9/l, dependent on additional risk factors for thrombosis and bleeding).
4 Also give for 3 weeks before and 4 weeks after elective DC cardioversion with target INR 2.5–3.0.
5 Dilated cardiomyopathy, mural thrombus post-MI or rheumatic valve disease.
6 Only for first 3–6 months post-insertion at discretion of each centre.

Although not yet in the BCSH guidelines, a target INR of 2.5 is widely agreed for nephrotic syndrome (generally, once albumin <25 g/l).

Starting Rx

Check INR before 1st dose and every day for 1st week, then assess stability of INR and scale down sensibly from loading regimen. If on heparin, do not stop until 2 days after therapeutic INR achieved.

For loading regimens, where possible use your hospital's own guidelines, since these often vary. Otherwise, it is sensible to use the BCSH guidelines:

Warfarin loading regimen. Adapted with permission of BMJ group from Fennerty, A. et al. *British Medical Journal* 1984; **288**: 1268–70.

Day 1		Day 2		Day 3		Day 4	
INR	Dose (mg)	INR	Dose (mg)	INR	Dose (mg)	INR	Dose* (mg)
<1.4	10	<1.8	10	<2.0	10	<1.4	>8
		1.8	1	2.0–2.1	5	1.4	8
		>1.8	0.5	2.2–2.3	4.5	1.5	7.5
				2.4–2.5	4	1.6–1.7	7
				2.6–2.7	3.5	1.8	6.5
				2.8–2.9	3	1.9	6
				3.0–3.1	2.5	2.0–2.1	5.5
				3.2–3.3	2	2.2–2.3	5
				3.4	1.5	2.4–2.6	4.5
				3.5	1	2.7–3.0	4
				3.6–4.0	0.5	3.1–3.5	3.5
				>4.0	0	3.6–4.0	3
						4.1–4.5	Miss 1 day then 2 mg
						>4.5	Miss 2 days then 1 mg

*Predicted maintenance dose.

> *Situations when doses (especially loading) may need review*
> ↓**doses if**: age >80 years, LF, HF, post-op, ↑baseline INR or taking drugs that potentiate warfarin (check for **W+** symbols in this book).
> ↑**doses if**: taking drugs that inhibit warfarin (check for **W−** symbols in this book).

Herbal remedies: can have significant interactions – always ask patients directly if taking any, as they may not realise the importance. Check each one with your hospital's drug information office for significance. Also beware glucosamine can ↑INR.
Alcohol and diet: can affect dosing, especially if intake varies – the goalposts will move for an individual's therapeutic range.
It is a common misconception that BMI influences response.

NB: there is evidence that loading with 5 mg for the 1st 3 days achieves therapeutic levels as quickly with less overshoot, and practice may soon change to reflect this. The latest British Society for Haematology guidelines (due for review in 2004) can be viewed at www.bcshguidelines.com.

If interrupting warfarin (e.g. before operation/procedure), do not reload post-op as above, but restart at double usual dose for 2 days, then return to usual dose *if no contraindications* (e.g. bleeding/taking **W+** drugs).

Make small infrequent dose changes unless INR dangerously high or low. 'Steering a supertanker' is a good analogy; there is often significant delay between dose changes and their fx.

Warfarin and surgery
Warfarin is often stopped 4–5 days ahead of surgery and other invasive procedures (±heparin cover until day of procedure). Exact protocol depends on procedure involved and risks of coming off warfarin: get senior advice from team doing the procedure ±haematologists if at all unsure.

Warfarin and pregnancy
Warfarin is contraindicated in early pregnancy (teratogenic during weeks 6–12). Women of childbearing age must be warned of potential risks/to seek haematology advice if planning pregnancy.

Overtreatment/poisoning

> *Seek expert help from haematology on-call* as xs vitamin K can make re-anticoagulation difficult, as fx can last for weeks ∴ ⇒ ↑risk from condition that warfarin was started for.

Recommendations for Mx of excess warfarin (BCSH guidelines). Adapted with permission from *British Journal of Haematology* 1998; **101**: 374–87 BCSM 2005 updates.

INR	Action
3.0–6.0 if target 2.5 (4.0–6.0 if target 3.5)	• ↓dose or stop warfarin; restart when INR <5.0
6.0–8.0 and no/minor bleeding	• Stop warfarin; restart when INR <5.0
>8.0 and no/minor bleeding	• Stop warfarin; restart when INR <5.0 • If other bleeding risks (e.g. age >70 yrs, Hx of bleeding complications *or* liver disease) give phytomenadione (vit K₁) 0.5 mg iv *or* 5 mg po
Major bleeding, e.g. ↓ing Hb or cardiodynamic instability	• Stop warfarin • Phytomenadione (vit K₁) 5 or 10 mg iv, repeating 24 h later if necessary • Prothrombin complex concentrate 30–50 units/kg (if unavailable give FFP 15 ml/kg)

HEPARIN

For immediate and short-term Rx/Px of TE. Two major types: low-molecular-weight heparins and unfractionated heparin.

Low-molecular-weight heparins (LMWHs)

Given sc. ↑Convenience (↓monitoring, can give to outpatients). ↓Incidence of HIT* and osteoporosis cf unfractionated heparin means now preferred for most indications (esp MI/ACS, DVT/PE, Rx and pre-cardioversion of AF). Dalteparin (Fragmin), enoxaparin (Clexane) and tinzaparin (Innohep) are the most commonly used; each hospital tends to use one in particular; ask nurses which one they stock or call pharmacy.

Monitoring
Via anti-Xa assay: usually necessary only if renal impairment (i.e. creatinine >150), pregnancy or at extremes of Wt (i.e. <45 kg or >100 kg). Take sample 3–4 h post dose.

> HIT* = heparin-induced thrombocytopoenia. It is not uncommon and can occur with all heparins. Watch for ↓ing platelet count. Get senior help if concerned. If confirmed, stop heparin immediately.

Unfractionated heparin

Given iv*: quickly reversible (immediately if protamine given; see p. 177), which makes it useful in settings where desired amount of anticoagulation may change rapidly, e.g. perioperatively, if patient at ↑risk of bleeding, or if using extracorporeal circuits such as cardiopulmonary bypass and haemodialysis. Also used with recombinant fibrinolytics in AMI.

   Can be given sc (only for Px), but now largely replaced by LMWH.

Monitoring
Via APTT ratio (=**A**ctivated **P**artial **T**hromboplastin **T**ime of patient divided by that of control serum). APTT is less commonly called KCCT. Results can (rarely) be given as patient's exact APTT: the normal range is 35–45 s. You then need to calculate the ratio: take the middle of the normal range of (i.e. 40 s) for your calculations. *Target ratio is commonly 1.5–2.5, but this can vary: check your hospital's protocol and aim for the middle of range.*
NB: there is no national (let alone international) consensus on methods of measuring APTT, so results are not yet standardised.

Starting iv treatment
1 *Load with 5000** units as iv bolus*: prescribed on the 'once-only' section of the drug chart (give 10 000** units if severe PE).
2 Set up ivi at 15–25 units/kg/h: usually = 1000–2000 units/h. A sensible starting rate is 1500 units/h, which can be achieved by

adding 25 000 units of heparin to 48 ml of normal saline to make 50 ml of solution (500 units/ml), which runs at 3 ml/h via a syringe driver. This can be written up as follows:

DATE/ TIME	INFUSION FLUID	VOLUME	ADDITIVES IF ANY DRUG AND DOSE	RATE OF ADMIN	DURA- TION	DR'S SIGNATURE	TIME START- ED	TIME COM- PLETED	SET UP BY SIG- NATURE	BATCH No.
08/01	Normal saline	50 ml	Heparin 25,000 units			TN				
	run at 3 ml per hour as ivi									

Figure 8 Drug chart, showing how to write up heparin infusion.

NB: dosing for co-therapy with fibrinolytics (according to ESC guidelines) is slightly different; see p. 179.

Check APTT ratio after every 6 h, then every 6–10 h until stable, and then daily at a minimum, adjusting to the following regimen:

APTT ratio	Action
<1.2	Give 5000-unit bolus iv and ↑ivi by 200–250 units/h
1.2–1.5	Give 2500-unit bolus iv and ↑ivi by 100–150 units/h
1.5–2.5	No change
2.5–3.0	↓ivi by 100–150 units/h
>3.0	Stop ivi for 1 h then restart ivi, ↓ing by 200–250 units/h

This regimen is based on APTT *ratio* therapeutic range of 1.5–2.5. *Don't take sample from drip arm* (unless from site distal to ivi).

Adjustments are safest made by writing a fresh ivi prescription at a different strength, but the same effect can also be achieved by calculating the appropriate rate change to the original prescription.

Variable rate of ivi (for fixed prescription of 25 000 units heparin in 50 ml saline)

Desired heparin ivi rate (units/h)	Rate of ivi (ml/h)	Desired heparin ivi rate (units/h)	Rate of ivi (ml/h)
1000	2.0	1500	3.0
1050	2.1	1550	3.1
1100	2.2	1600	3.2
1150	2.3	1650	3.3
1200	2.4	1700	3.4
1250	2.5	1750	3.5
1300	2.6	1800	3.6
1350	2.7	1850	3.7
1400	2.8	1900	3.8
1450	2.9	1950	3.9

Overtreatment/poisoning (all heparins)
If significant bleeding, stop heparin and observe: iv heparin has short $t_{1/2}$ (30 min–2 h), so fx wear off quickly. If bleeding continues or is life-threatening, consider iv protamine (1 mg per 80–100 units of heparin to be neutralised as ivi over 10 min. ↓doses if giving >15 min after heparin stopped). NB: protamine is less effective against LMWH, and repeat administration may be required.
   Seek expert help from haematology on-call if in any doubt!

THROMBOLYSIS

INDICATIONS

From Resuscitation Council (UK) guidelines 2005.

- Onset of chest pain <12 h + Hx compatible with MI + one of:
  - ST elevation ≥2 mV (=2 small squares) in ≥2 adjacent chest leads
  - ST elevation ≥1 mV (=1 small square) in ≥2 limb leads
  - new LBBB: must assume it is new if cannot prove is old

- Onset of chest pain 12–24 h ago and evidence of an evolving infarct, e.g. ongoing chest pain or worsening ECG changes.

NB: Posterior infarcts are also widely considered to be an indication for thrombolysis. Diagnosis can be hard (look for ST depression + dominant R wave in V1–3); get cardiology advice if suspicious.

> Treatment needs to be started ASAP as 'time = myocardium' and 'door to needle time' is important. Out-of-hospital thromobolysis (e.g. by paramedics) saves time (about 1 h) and its use is ↑ing.

☠CONTRAINDICATIONS☠

From ESC guidelines 2003 (with permission from *European Heart Journal* 2003; **24**: 28–66). Local guidelines/checklists often exist and should be used if available: consult cardiology ± haematology on-call if in any doubt.

Absolute
- Haemorrhagic stroke or stroke of unknown origin at any time.
- Ischaemic stroke in preceding 6 months.
- CNS damage or neoplasms.
- Major trauma/surgery/head injury in preceding 3 weeks.
- GI bleeding within the last month.
- Known bleeding disorder.
- Aortic dissection.

Relative
- TIA in past 6 months.
- Oral anticoagulant therapy.
- Pregnancy or within 1 week postpartum.
- Non-compressible punctures.
- Traumatic resuscitation.
- Refractory hypertension (systolic >180 mmHg).
- Advanced liver disease.
- Infective endocarditis.
- Active peptic ulcer.

CHOICE OF AGENT

Always use your hospital's protocol if one exists – contact CCU, A&E or look on your hospital intranet for details.

Choose between streptokinase and a recombinant thrombolytic such as alteplase, reteplase or tenecteplase (each hospital tends to stock one in particular).

NICE guidance recommends that, in hospitals, the choice of agent should take account of:

- *'The likely balance of benefit and harm (e.g. stroke) to which each of the thrombolytic agents would expose the individual patient.'* Recombinant forms (compared with streptokinase) are probably more efficacious and have ↓incidence of allergic reactions, CCF and bleeding other than stroke. However they have ↑incidence of haemorrhagic stroke.
- *'Current UK clinical practice, in which it is accepted that patients who have previously received streptokinase should not be treated with it again.'* Streptokinase is less effective and more likely to cause allergic reaction after first administration (due to Ab production). Don't give if patient has been given it in the past.
- *'The hospital's arrangements for reducing delays in the administration of thrombolysis.'* Some agents are quicker to set up and administer and this can reduce 'door to needle times'.

Heparin co-therapy
Recombinant forms always need concurrent iv heparin for 24–48 h (this does not usually apply for *streptokinase*). Use your hospital's A&E/CCU protocol if one exists. Otherwise use *ESC guidelines*: 60 units/kg (max 4000 units) iv bolus, then ivi at 12 units/kg/h for 24–48 h (max 1000 units/h). Monitor APTT at 3, 6, 12, 24 and 48 h, with target APTT (≠ APTT *ratio*!) of 50–70 s. NB: this is different to 'standard' iv heparin regimens (see pp. 175–7).

Side effects

Commonly bleeding (mostly mild and at iv sites; if severe or suspect CVA, stop ivi and get senior help), N&V, ↓BP (improves if transiently ↓ rate of ivi and raise legs), mild hypersensitivity (inc uveitis). Rarely anaphylaxis, GBS.

CONTROLLED DRUGS

In the UK special 'Prescription requirements' apply to 'Schedule' 1, 2 or 3 drugs only, the most likely of which to be prescribed by junior doctors are morphine, diamorphine, fentanyl, methadone, (& less commonly buprenorphine or pethidine). These requirements don't apply to codeine, dihydrocodeine (including DF118), tramadol or benzodiazepines. For full details on controlled drug guidance in the UK see www.dh.gov.uk/controlleddrugs.

  The following must be written in the *doctor's own handwriting*:

* Date: may be stamped but *not* computer-generated.
* Full name and address of patient.
* Drug name plus its form* (and, where appropriate, strength).
* Dosing regimen.
* Total amount of drug to be dispensed *in words and figures*.
* Prescribers address must be specified (should already be on prescription form).

  *Omitting the form is a common reason for an invalid prescription. It is often assumed to be obvious from the prescription (e.g. fentanyl as a patch or Oramorph as a liquid), but it still has to be written.

Miscellaneous

INTRAVENOUS FLUIDS

CRYSTALLOIDS

Isotonic: used mostly for maintenance (replacement) regimens:

- *Normal (0.9%) saline:* 1 litre contains 150 mmol Na^+.
- *5% glucose*:* 1 litre contains 278 mmol (=50 g) glucose, which is immediately metabolised and included only to make the fluid isotonic (calories are minimal, at 220 kcal). Used as method of giving pure H_2O and as ivi with insulin sliding scales (see p. 168).
- *Glucose* saline:* 1 litre contains mixture of NaCl (30 mmol Na^+) and glucose (4% = 222 mmol). Useful as contains correct proportions of constituents (excluding KCl, which can be added to each bag) for average daily requirements (see below). Suboptimal long term, as does not account for individual patient needs (esp if these are far from average). Also used as ivi in insulin sliding scales (see pp. 168–9).

Non-isotonic: used less commonly; mostly specialist situations only:

- *Hypertonic (5%) saline:* 1 litre contains 750 mmol Na^+; given mostly for severe hyponatraemia. ☠Seek specialist help first.☠
- *Hypotonic (0.45%) saline:* for severe ↑Na^+ (e.g. HONK).
- *10% and 20% glucose*:* for mild/moderate hypoglycaemia.
- *50% glucose:* for severe hypoglycaemia (see p. 206) and if insulin being used to lower K^+ (see p. 209).

*NB: glucose = dextrose. Low-strength glucose solutions used to be called dextrose solutions; this is now being phased out.

COLLOIDS (= plasma substitutes/expanders)

- Gelofusine: gelatin-based and used in resuscitation of shock (non-cardiogenic). NB: the electrolyte contents are often overlooked: 1 litre Gelofusine has 154 mmol Na^+.
- *Hartmann's solution:* compound sodium lactate, used in surgery/trauma (also 1 litre contains 5 mmol K^+).

STANDARD DAILY REQUIREMENTS

= 3 litres H_2O, 40–70 mmol K^+, 100–150 mmol Na^+.

If no oral intake (preoperative, $\downarrow$GCS, unsafe swallow, post-CVA, etc.), this can be provided as follows:

DATE	INFUSION FLUID	VOL-UME	ADDITIVES IF ANY DRUG AND DOSE	RATE OF ADMIN	DURA-TION	DR'S SIGNATURE	TIME START-ED	TIME COM-PLETED	SET UP BY SIG-NATURE	BATCH No.
08/01	5% Glucose	1 litre	20 mmol KCl		8h	TN				
08/01	Normal saline	1 litre			8h	TN				
08/01	5% Glucose	1 litre	20 mmol KCl		8h	TN				

Figure 9 Drug chart, showing how to write up intravenous fluids.

This '2 sweet (5% glucose), 1 sour (0.9% saline)' regimen is commonly used in fit preoperative patients. If in any doubt, normal (0.9%) saline is generally safest, unless liver failure (see below) or if Na^+ outside normal range ($\downarrow$ or $\uparrow$). Always get senior help if unsure: incorrect fluids can be as dangerous as any other drug.

Individual requirements may differ substantially according to:

- Body habitus, age, residual oral intake, if on multiple iv drugs (which are sometimes given with significant amounts of fluid).
- Insensible losses (normally about 1 litre/day). $\uparrow$skin losses if fever or burns. $\uparrow$lung losses in hyperventilation or inhalation burns.
- GI losses (normally about 0.2 litre/day). Any vomiting ($\uparrow Cl^-$ content) or diarrhoea ($\uparrow K^+$ content) must be taken into account as well as less obvious causes, e.g. ileus, fistulae.
- Fluid compartment shifts, esp vasodilation if sepsis/anaphylaxis.

All the above points seem obvious but are easy to forget!

K^+ CONSIDERATIONS

Do not give >10 mmol/h unless K^+ dangerously low, when it can be given quicker (see p. 209). Surgical patients often need less K^+ in

1st 24 h post-op, as K^+ is released by cell death ($\therefore$ proportional to extent of surgery).

IMPORTANT POINTS

- *Take extreme care if major organ failure:*
  - *Heart failure:* heart can quickly become 'overloaded' and $\Rightarrow$ acute LVF. Even if not currently in HF, beware if predisposed (e.g. Hx of HF or IHD).
  - *Renal failure:* unless pre-renal cause (e.g. hypovolaemia), do not give more fluid than residual renal function can deal with. Seek help from renal team if at all concerned; good fluid Mx greatly influences outcomes in this group.
  - *Liver failure: **should not receive any saline**;* always use 5% glucose. Serum Na^+ may be $\downarrow$d, but total body Na^+ is often $\uparrow$d. Any saline will work its way into the wrong compartment (e.g. peritoneal fluid $\therefore$ $\uparrow$ing ascites).
- If in doubt, give 'fluid challenges': small volumes (normally 200–500 ml) of fluid over short periods of time, to see whether clinical response to BP, urine output or left verticular function is beneficial or detrimental before committing to longer-term fluid strategy.
- In general, encourage oral fluids: homeostasis (if normal) is safer, less expensive and less consuming of doctor/nurse time than iv fluids. Beware if $\downarrow$swallow, fluid overload (esp if HF or RF), pre-/post-operative or if homeostasis disorders (esp SIADH).
- Check the following before prescribing any iv fluids:
  - *Clinical markers of hydration:* skin turgor/temperature, mucous membranes, JVP, peripheral oedema, pulmonary oedema. Often overlooked and very useful!
  - *Recent input and output:* if at all concerned, ask nurses for strict fluid balance chart. Daily weights are often very informative, esp if doubts over accuracy of fluid charts.
  - Recent U&Es, esp K^+.

It can be difficult to illicit all this information under time pressure. The trick is to know when to take extreme care. Be particularly careful if you do not know the patient when on call, and be wary when asked to 'just write up another bag' without reviewing the patient. Often, you will be asked to prescribe fluids when no longer necessary or even when they may be harmful. To save time for those on call (and to $\uparrow$ the chances of your patients getting appropriate fluids), leave clear instructions with the nurses and on the drug chart for as long as can be sensibly predicted (esp over weekends/long holidays).

STEROIDS

CORTICOSTEROIDS

The most commonly used systemic drugs are:

Drug	Equivalent dose	Main uses
Prednisolone	5 mg	Acute asthma/COPD, rheumatoid arthritis (po)
Methylprednisolone	4 mg	Acute flares rheumatoid arthritis/MS (iv)
Dexamethasone	750 µg	$\uparrow$ICP, CAH, Dx Cushing's (iv/po)
Hydrocortisone	20 mg	Acute asthma/COPD (iv)

Glucocorticoid fx predominate; mineralocorticoid fx for these are all mild apart from hydrocortisone (has moderate fx) and dexamethasone (has minimal fx $\therefore$ used when H_2O and Na^+ retention are particularly undesirable, e.g. $\uparrow$ICP).

Side effects = Cushing's syndrome!
- *Metabolic:* Na^+/fluid retention*, hyperlipoproteinaemia, leukocytosis, negative K^+/Ca^{2+}/nitrogen balance, generalised fluid/electrolyte abnormalities.
- *Endocrine:* hyperglycaemia/$\downarrow$GTT (can $\Rightarrow$ DM), adrenal suppression.
  - *Fat*:* truncal obesity, moon face, interscapular ('buffalo hump') and suprascapular fat pads.

- *Skin:* hirsutism, bruising/purpura, acne, striae, ↓healing, telangiectasia, thinning.
  - *Other:* impotence, menstrual irregularities/amenorrhoea, ↓growth (children), ↑appetite*.
- *GI:* pancreatitis, peptic/oesophageal ulcers: give PPI if on ↑doses.
- *Cardiac:* HTN, CCF, myocardial rupture post-MI, TE.
- *Musculoskeletal:* proximal myopathy, osteoporosis, fractures (can ⇒ avascular necrosis).
- *Neurological:* ↑epilepsy, ↑ICP/papilloedema (esp children on withdrawal of corticosteroids).
- *Ψ:* mood Δs (↑ or ↓), psychosis (esp at ↑doses), dependence.
- *Ocular:* cataracts, glaucoma, corneal/scleral thinning.
- *Infections:* ↑susceptibility, ↑speed (↑severity at presentation), TB reactivation, ↑risk of chickenpox/shingles/measles.

> SEs are dose-dependent. If patient is on high doses, make sure this is intentional: it is not rare in fluctuating (e.g. inflammatory) illnesses for patient to be left on high doses by mistake. Seek specialist advice if unsure.

Cautions

Can mostly be worked out from the SEs. Caution should be taken if patient already has a condition that is a potential SE. Systemic corticosteroids are CI in systemic infections (w/o antibiotic cover). NB: avoid live vaccines. If never had chickenpox, avoid exposure.

Interactions

Apply to all systemic Rx. fx can be ↓d by rifampicin, carbamazepine, phenytoin and phenobarbital. fx can be ↑d by erythromycin, ketoconazole, itraconazole and ciclosporin (whose own fx are ↑d by methylprednisolone). ↑risk of ↓K⁺ with amphotericin and digoxin.

Withdrawal effects

Acute adrenal insufficiency (= Addisonian crisis; 💀can be fatal💀 see p. 208), ↓BP, fever, myalgia, arthralgia, rhinitis, conjunctivitis, painful itchy nodules, ↓Wt. ∴ must withdraw slowly if patient has had >3 wks Rx (or a shorter course w/in 1 year of stopping long-term Rx), other causes of adrenal suppression, received high doses (>40 mg od prednisolone or equivalent), or repeat doses in evening, or repeat course. Also note intercurrent illness, trauma, surgery needs ↑doses and can precipitate relative withdrawal.

Steroid Rx card must be carried by all patients on prolonged Rx.

MINERALOCORTICOIDS e.g. fludrocortisone

Used for Addison's disease and acute adrenocortical deficiency (rarely needed for hypopituitarism). Can also be used for orthostatic/postural hypotension. Main SEs are H_2O/Na^+ retention.

SEDATION/SLEEPING TABLETS

ACUTE SEDATION/RAPID TRANQUILLISATION

For the acutely agitated, disturbed or violent patient (and for temporary sedation before unpleasant procedures).

Important points
- Organic causes are commonest cause outside of Ψ wards: look for and treat sepsis, hypoxia, drug withdrawal (esp alcohol/opiates) and metabolic causes (esp hypoglycaemia).
- A well-lit calm room and reassurance can be all that is required.
- Oral medications should be tried first if possible.
- Obtain as much drug Hx as possible, esp of antipsychotics and benzodiazepines as influences selection of appropriate agent/dose.

There are two main choices: antipsychotics and benzodiazepines: ☺ good for/reasons to choose; ☹ bad for/reasons to not give.

Antipsychotics
☺ Taking benzodiazepines, elderly or psychotic features (e.g. Schneiderian 1st-rank symptoms or Hx of schizophrenia).
☹ Antipsychotic-naive, alcohol withdrawal, cardiac disease, movement disorders (esp Parkinson's; extrapyramidal fx (see pp. 192–3) are common – treat with procyclidine).

- *Haloperidol* 0.5–5 mg po (or im if necessary). 2.5 mg is sensible starting dose for delirium in elderly. 5 mg is safe for acute psychosis in young adults. Maximum 18 mg im or 30 mg po in 24 h (write up prn).
- If suspect *acute schizophrenia*, NICE guidelines now recommend atypical antipsychotic as 1st-line, e.g. olanzapine 10 mg po (⇒ ↓SEs) – now also available im.

Benzodiazepines

☺ Alcohol withdrawal, anxiety, at night time (are 'hypnotic').
☹ Respiratory disease (esp COPD/asthma), elderly (⇒ falls and rarely paradoxical agitation/aggression).

- *Lorazepam* 0.5–1 mg po/im/iv (maximum 4 mg/24 h). Shorter acting than diazepam ∴ better if hepatic impairment.
- *Diazepam* 2–5 mg po/iv (if iv preferably as Diazemuls) or 10–20 mg pr. ↑doses if tolerance/much previous exposure to benzodiazepines.
- *Midazolam* 1.0–7.5 mg iv: titrate up slowly, according to response. Requires iv access and is used mostly for cooperative patients ahead of unpleasant procedures (less suitable for very agitated patients). Also wears off relatively quickly.

SLEEPING TABLETS

Try to avoid giving:

- for >2–4 wks (dependency common). Try reassurance/↑'sleep hygiene'/non-pharmacological measures 1st. Treat depression if 1° cause
- at all if hepatic encephalopathy or ↓respiratory reserve (esp asthma/COPD; NB: *hypoxia can also ⇒ restlessness and agitation!*).

Choose from:

1. Benzodiazepines: ↑ the major inhibitory neurotransmitter GABA via their own (benzodiazepine) receptor.

- *Temazepam* 10 mg nocte (can ↑ to 20 mg).

Halve doses if LF (avoid if severe; consider oxazepam or lorazepam instead), RF or elderly.

2. 'Z'/Benzodiazepine-like drugs: similarly ↑s GABA.

- *Zopiclone* 7.5 mg nocte.
- *Zolpidem* 10 mg nocte.
- *Zaleplon* 10 mg nocte.

Halve doses if LF (avoid if severe), RF or elderly.

3. Sedating antihistamines: are a good alternative: ⇒ ↓respiratory depression/addiction but ↑hangover drowsiness; effectiveness may ↓ after several days of Rx ∴ good for inpatients as short-term Rx.

- *Promethazine* 25 mg nocte (can ↑dose to 50 mg)

BENZODIAZEPINES

Varying pharmacokinetics are utilised. If shorter-acting,
⇒ ↓hangover/drowsiness (and ↓accumulation in LF) but
⇒ ↑withdrawal fx when stopped.

ADVERSE EFFECTS

> ☠*Respiratory depression*☠
> Especially in elderly and if naive to benzodiazepines. Put on close nursing observations and monitor O₂ sats if concerned. If using very high doses, get iv access and have flumazenil at hand.

- *Dependence/tolerance:* common ∴ prescribe long-term benzodiazepines *only if absolutely necessary* and withdraw ASAP. In order to withdraw safely, if not already on one, swap to long-acting drug (e.g. diazepam) and take 1/8 off the dose every 2 weeks. Try β-blockers to reduce anxiety (avoid antipsychotics).
- *Withdrawal symptoms:* rebound insomnia, tremor, anxiety, confusion, anorexia, toxic psychosis, convulsions, sweating.

Comparison of commonly used benzodiazepines; adapted from www.benzo.org.uk (an excellent resource for information on benzodiazepines), with permission from Professor C.H. Ashton, Institute of Neuroscience, University of Newcastle, UK.

$t_{1/2}$(h)[1]	Drug	Equivalent dose (mg)[1]	Main use(s)
2–3	Midazolam	N/A	Temporary sedation for procedures (titrated iv)
4–15	Oxazepam	20	Good in LF (↓accumulation of metabolites)
6–12	Alprazolam[2]	0.5	Anxiety
6–12	Loprazolam[2]	1–2	Anxiety, insomnia
8–20	Lorazepam	1	Status epilepticus (iv), acute ψ sedation (im/po)
8–22	Temazepam	20	Insomnia
12–60	Clobazam	20	Epilepsy, anxiety
18–50	Clonazepam	0.5	Movement disorders, epilepsy and ψ disorders
36–200[3]	Diazepam	10	Status epilepticus (iv/pr), anxiety, alcohol withdrawal
36–200[3]	Chlordiazepoxide	25	Alcohol withdrawal

[1]These are approximate and can vary considerably between individuals. [2]Rarely used in the UK.
[3]These values are for the *active metabolite*.

SIDE-EFFECT PROFILES

Knowledge of these, together with a drug's mechanism(s), will simplify learning and allow anticipation of drug SEs.

CHOLINOCEPTORS

ACh stimulates nicotinic and muscarinic receptors. Anticholinesterases ⇒ ↑ACh and ∴ stimulate both receptor types and have 'cholinergic fx'. Drugs that ↓cholinoceptor action do so mostly via muscarinic receptors (antinicotinics used only in anaesthesia) and are ∴ more accurately called 'antimuscarinics' rather than 'anticholinergics'.

Cholinergic fx	Antimuscarinic fx
Generally ↑*secretions*	*Generally* ↓*secretions*
Diarrhoea	**C**onstipation
Urination	**U**rinary retention
Miosis (constriction)	**M**ydriasis/↓accommodation*
Bronchospasm/**B**radycardia**	**B**ronchodilation/Tachycardia
Excitation of CNS (and muscle)	**D**rowsiness, **D**ry eyes, **D**ry skin
Lacrimation ↑	
Saliva/**S**weat ↑	
Commonly caused by:	
Anticholinesterases:	Atropine, ipratropium (Atrovent)
MG Rx, e.g. pyridostigmine	Antihistamines (inc cyclizine)
Dementia Rx, e.g. rivastigmine, donepezil	Antidepressants (esp TCAs)
	Antipsychotics (esp 'typicals')
	Hyoscine, Ia antiarrhythmics

*⇒ blurred vision and ↑IOP. **Together with vasodilation ⇒ ↓BP.

ADRENOCEPTORS

α *generally excites sympathetic system (except*):*

$\alpha_1 \Rightarrow$ GI smooth-muscle relaxation*, otherwise contracts smooth muscle: vasoconstriction, GI/bladder sphincter constriction (uterus, seminal tract, iris (radial muscle)). Also ↑salivary secretion, ↓glycogenolysis (in liver).

$\alpha_2 \Rightarrow$ inhibition of neurotransmitters (esp NA and ACh for feedback control), Pt aggregation, contraction of vascular smooth muscle, inhibition of insulin release. Also prominent adrenoceptor of CNS (inhibits sympathetic outflow).

β *generally inhibits sympathetic system (except*):*

$\beta_1 \Rightarrow$ ↑HR*, ↑contractility* (and ↑s salivary amylase secretion).

$\beta_2 \Rightarrow$ Vasodilation, bronchodilation, muscle tremor, glycogenolysis (in hepatic and skeletal muscle). Also ↑s renin secretion, relaxes ciliary muscle and visceral smooth muscles (GI sphincter, bladder detrusor, uterus if not pregnant).

$\beta_3 \Rightarrow$ lipolysis, thermogenesis (of little pharmacological relevance).

SEROTONIN (5HT)

Relative excess: 'serotonin syndrome'; seen with antidepressants at ↑doses or if swapped without adequate 'tapering' or 'washout period'. Initially causes restlessness, sweating and tremor, progressing to shivering, myoclonus and confusion, and, if severe enough, convulsions/death.

Relative deficit: 'antidepressant withdrawal/discontinuation syndrome' occurs when antidepressants stopped too quickly; likelihood depends on $t_{1/2}$ of drug. Causes ''flu-like' symptoms (chills/sweating, myalgia, headache and nausea), shock-like sensations, dizziness, anxiety, irritability, insomnia, vivid dreams. Rarely ⇒ movement disorders and ↓memory/concentration.

DOPAMINE (DA)

Relative excess: causes behaviour Δ, confusion and psychosis (esp if predisposed, e.g. schizophrenia). Seen with L-dopa and DA agonists used in Parkinson's (and some endocrine disorders), e.g. bromocriptine.

Relative deficit: causes extrapyramidal fx (see below), ↑prolactin (sexual dysfunction, female infertility, gynaecomastia), neuroleptic malignant syndrome. Seen with DA antagonists, esp antipsychotics and certain antiemetics such as metoclopramide, prochlorperazine and levomepromazine.

EXTRAPYRAMIDAL EFFECTS

Abnormalities of movement control arising from dysfunction of basal ganglia.

- *Parkinsonism:* rigidity and bradykinesia ± tremor.
- *Dyskinesias* (= abnormal involuntary movements): commonly:
  - *Dystonia* (= abnormal posture): dynamic (e.g. oculogyric crisis) or static (e.g. torticollis).
  - *Tardive (delayed onset) dyskinesia:* esp orofacial movements.
  - *Others:* tremor, chorea, athetosis, hemiballismus, myoclonus, tics.
- *Akathisia* (= restlessness): esp after large antipsychotic doses.

All are commonly caused by antipsychotics (esp older 'typical' drugs) and are a rare complication of antiemetics (e.g. metoclopramide, prochlorperazine – esp in young women). Dyskinesias and dystonias are common with antiparkinsonian drugs (esp peaks of L-dopa doses).

Most respond to stopping (or ↓dose of) the drug – if not possible, doesn't work or immediate Rx needed add antimuscarinic drug (e.g. procyclidine) but doesn't work for akithisia (try β-blocker) and can worsen tardive dyskinesia: seek neurology ± psychiatry opinion if in doubt.

CEREBELLAR EFFECTS

Esp antiepileptics (e.g. phenytoin) and alcohol.

- **D**ysdiadokokinesis, dysmetria (= past-pointing) and rebound.
- **A**taxia of gait (wide-based, irregular step length) ± trunk.
- **N**ystagmus: towards side of lesion; mostly coarse and horizontal.
- **I**ntention tremor (also titubation = nodding-head tremor).
- **S**peech: scanning dysarthria – slow, slurred or jerky.
- **H**ypotonia (less commonly hyporeflexia or pendular reflexes).

CYTOCHROME P450

Important inhibitors	Important inducers
Heart/liver failure	Cigarettes
Omeprazole	**P**henytoin
Fluoxetine/**F**luconazole	**C**arbamazepine
Disulfiram	**B**arbiturates (e.g. phenobarbital)
Erythromycin and clarithromycin	**R**ifampicin
Valproate	**A**lcohol (chronic abuse*)
Isoniazid	**S**ulphonylureas/**St** John's wort
Cimetidine/**C**iprofloxacin	
EtOH (acute abuse – note *chronic* abuse can induce!*)	
Sulphonamides	

Substrates of P450 that often result in significant interactions (these drugs can ⇒ severe problems if rendered ineffective or toxic by interactions ∴ always exclude interactions when prescribing!):

- Inhibitors and inducers can affect warfarin, phenytoin carbamazepine, ciclosporin and theophyllines. Interactions can ∴ ⇒ toxicity **or** treatment failure.
- Inducers affect OCP ∴ can ⇒ failure as contraceptive!

NB: This system is very complex and mediated by many isoenzymes; predicting significant interactions requires understanding which drugs are metabolised by which isoenzymes as well as which, and to what degree, other drugs effect these isoenzymes. Look for **P450** symbols in this book as a rough guide; check SPCs if concerned (available online at www.emc.medicines.org.uk) and for a full overview of the **P450** system see www.edhayes.com/startp450.html

Medical emergencies

This section is intended only as a reminder/checklist. It is not a complete guide to Mx, which can be found in other sources and online (e.g. www.eboncall.org). Local Rx preferences and individuality of patients/diseases mean that it is impossible to outline the perfect Rx for every occasion: *always seek senior help if unsure!*
☠ In all emergencies, first follow *ABC + Disability (GCS)* ± *Exposure*. Obtain as much Hx and perform as much examination as is possible. Take time to think and assess: it is more far more common that things go wrong due to a lack of thinking than lack of action. ☠

ACUTE CORONARY SYNDROMES (ACS)

Clues: angina, N&V, sweating, LVF (see p. 199), ↓BP, Hx of IHD. Remember atypical pain and silent infarcts in DM, elderly or if ↓GCS.

There are three acute coronary syndromes:

1. **STEMI:** ST Elevation Myocardial Infarction (see pp. 177–8).
2. **NSTEMI:** Non-ST Elevation MI; troponin (T or I) +ve.
3. **UA(P):** Unstable Angina (Pectoris); troponin (T or I) −ve

FOR ALL ACS

- O_2: maximal flow through re-breather mask (care if COPD).
- *Aspirin*: 300 mg po stat (chew/dispersible form) unless CI. If in A&E, check has not given already by paramedics or GP.
- *Clopidogrel*: 300 mg po (some give 600 mg, esp if immediate PCI planned).
- *Opiate*: in UK most centres give diamorphine 2.5–5 mg iv +antiemetic (e.g. metoclopramide 10 mg iv), repeat diamorphine iv according to response. Morphine is an alternative, initially 3–5 mg iv, repeating every few minutes until pain free.
- *GTN*: 1–2 sprays or sl tablets (max 1.2 mg). If pain continues or LVF develops, set up ivi, titrating to BP and pain. NB: can ⇒ ↓BP; don't give if systolic ≤100 mmHg (esp if combined with ↓BP) or inferior infarct (i.e. suspected RV involvement).

DATE/ TIME	INFUSION FLUID	VOL- UME	ADDITIVES IF ANY DRUG AND DOSE	RATE OF ADMIN	DURA- TION	DR'S SIGNATURE	TIME START- ED	TIME COM- PLETED	SET UP BY SIG- NATURE	BATCH No.
25/12	N. Saline	50 ml	50 mg GTN	0-10 ml/hr*		TN				
	*TITRATE TO PAIN: Stop if systolic BP < 100 mmHg									

Figure 10 Drug chart, showing how to write up GTN ivi.

Consider:

- *β-blocker:* unless CI (see propranolol p. 109), esp beware ☠asthma, acute LVF☠, ↓BP (systolic <100 mmHg), ↓HR (<60/min), 2nd-/3rd-degree HB; get senior help if in doubt.
  - *Can be given iv or po:* it is often recommended to give iv for STEMI and po for NSTEMI and UAP. In acute settings, metoprolol is often drug of choice as short $t_{1/2}$ means it wears off quickly if LVF develops. Consult local protocol or get senior advice if unsure.
  - *iv:* e.g. metoprolol 1–5 mg iv, giving 1–2 mg aliquots at a time whilst monitoring BP and HR. Repeat to max 15 mg, stopping when BP ≤100 mmHg or HR ≤60. Then consider starting metoprolol po.
  - *po:* e.g. metoprolol 12.5–50 mg tds. If cardiodynamically stable 24 h later, change to long acting β-blocker, e.g. atenolol 50 mg od.
  - If already on β-blocker, ensure dose adequate to control HR.
  - If β-blocker CI and ↑HR consider Ca^{2+} blocker and get senior ± cardiology advice.
- *Insulin:* for all type I DM and type II DM or non-diabetics with CBG >11 on admission. Give conventional sliding scale or GIK ivi (e.g. DIGAMI) if local protocol exists; contact CCU for advice.
- *iv fluids:* if RV infarct. Clues: ↓BP with no pulmonary oedema, inferior or posterior ECG Δs (esp ST elevation ≥1 mm in a VF) and ↑JVP. If suspected, do right-sided ECG and look for ↑ST in V4. Avoid vasodilating drugs (esp nitrates and ACE-i). Care with β-blockers (can ⇒HB).

IF STEMI

- *Reperfusion therapy: primary PCI (if available) or thrombolysis.*
  NB: starting one or the other ASAP is paramount ('time = myocardium'!) ∴ if appropriate, initiate/organise during above steps. See pp. 177–80 for thrombolysis indications, CIs and choice of agent.
- *Heparin:* iv heparin is given with *recombinant* thrombolytics for 24–48 h (see p. 179) to avoid the rebound hypercoagulable states they can cause, but is *not* needed with *streptokinase*. If ongoing chest pain or ECG Δs, get senior advice on further anticoagulation; consider iv heparin if PCI a possibility, otherwise consider LMWH (e.g. enoxaparin 1 mg/kg bd sc or daltperin 120 units/kg bd sc) but must be balanced against ↑risk of intracranial haemorrhage if >75 yrs old.
- Consider (consult local protocol/cardiology on-call if unsure):
  - *Glycoprotein IIb/IIIa inhibitor:* esp if not thrombolysed (CI or presentation too late) or PCI planned and still unstable. Use with caution (esp <48 h post-thrombolysis).
  - Rescue PCI: esp if thrombolysis given and doesn't ↓pain/settle ECG Δs.

IF NSTEMI OR UAP

- *Heparin:* LMWH, e.g. enoxaparin 1 mg/kg bd sc or daltparin 120 units/kg bd sc. Consider iv heparin if PCI planned in 1st 24–36 h after symptom onset.
- Consider (consult local protocol/cardiology on-call if unsure):
  - *Glycoprotein IIb/IIIa inhibitor:* if high risk* (defined by ERC as: haemodynamic or rhythm instability, persistent pain, acute or dynamic ECG Δs, DM, ↑troponin) and/or ongoing chest pain/ECG Δs.

SECONDARY PREVENTION

For all ACS unless CI or already started:

- *Next day:* aspirin 75 mg od, 'statin' (e.g. simvastatin 20 mg od) and clopidogrel 75 mg od (for 1 yr[NICE]).
- *When stable:* β-blocker (if not already started, e.g. atenolol 50 mg od once any LVF clears; see above for CI) and ACE-i (e.g.

ramipril 2.5 mg bd po started 3–10 days after MI, then 5 mg bd after 2 days if tolerated).

- *ASAP:* diet/lifestyle Δs (↓Wt, diet Δs, ↑exercise, ↓smoking, etc.).

ACUTE LVF

Clues: SOB, S_3 or S_4, pulmonary oedema (can ⇒ pink frothy sputum if severe), Hx of IHD, ↑JVP (if also RVF, i.e. CCF).

- 60–100% O_2 (care if COPD) and sit patient upright.
- Furosemide 80 mg iv; consider repeat doses or ivi later. If not 'in extremis', consider ↓doses (40 or 60 mg).
- Diamorphine 2.5–5.0 mg iv + metoclopramide 10 mg iv.
- GTN ivi: see ACS section pp. 196–7.

If patient does not respond/worsens, get senior help and consider:

- *Non-invasive ventilation* (NIV) as continuous positive airways pressure (CPAP). If no machine on ward, find one ASAP!
- *Inotropes:* if ↓BP, e.g. dobutamine via central line; if patient is this sick, will also be needed for CVP measurement. Get senior help if needed.
- *?Underlying cause:* MI, arrhythmias (esp AF), ↑↑BP, ↓↓Hb, ARF, anaphylaxis, sepsis, ARDS, poisons/OD (e.g. aspirin).
- *ACE-i:* once stable and if no CI, e.g. enalapril 2.5 mg od (↑later).

ACCELERATED HYPERTENSION

Dx: diastolic ≥120 mmHg (or systolic ≥220 mmHg) **plus** grade III (haemorrhages/exudates) or IV (papilloedema) hypertensive retinopathy. ☠ Do not drop BP too quickly as can ⇒ MI, CVA or ARF. ☠ NB: patients are often salt and water deplete (look for postural drop of ≥20 mmHg) so *may require fluid replacement as well as antihypertensives.*

If life-threatening target organ damage (e.g. encephalopathy, intracranial haemorrhage, aortic dissection, unstable angina, acute MI, acute LVF/pulmonary oedema or pre-eclampsia/eclampsia): get senior help immediately and aim to ↓diastolic to 110–115 mmHg over 4–6 h and then more slowly thereafter (e.g. ↓diastolic to <100 mmHg after

48 h). This should **always** be done in the ITU/HDU/CCU setting and generally (but not always) involve *iv* antihypertensives; choose from nitroprusside (most commonly used but can ⇒ cyanide poisoning, esp if RF), hydralazine (commonly used in pregnancy), labetalol (safe in pregnancy but can ⇒ severe ↓BP) or phentolamine (esp if phaeo known/suspected). If pulmonary oedema, consider GTN/ISDN.

If no life-threatening target organ damage (i.e. renal failure, mild LVF etc): aim to ↓diastolic BP to 110–115 mmHg over 24–48 h using *oral* medication such as:

- *Nifedipine (e.g. Adalat) Retard* 10 mg po. Monitor and reassess; consider repeat doses (e.g. after 2 h) and if required/tolerated aiming to get patient on to higher doses (e.g. 20 mg tds). Tablets to be swallowed (not chewed) and avoid quick release or sl preparations. Convert to amlodipine once stable.
  - If IHD or ↑HR consider adding β-blocker* later (e.g. atenolol 25–50 mg od).
  - If nifedipine CI, consider β-blocker instead*: metoprolol is good choice (e.g. 12.5–25 mg initially then tds regimen) as short acting and needs no dose adjustment in RF. Consider converting to atenolol (e.g. 50 mg po) once stable.
  - Other drugs to consider are ACE-i (can ⇒ severe ↓BP; if so give iv saline) and diuretics (if patient fluid overloaded).

*Beware if cause is phaeo: will need α-blocker (e.g. phenoxybenzamine) and salt supplements. If tachycardia a problem, must not give β-blocker until several days after α-blocker started. Suspect if BP very variable, headaches, sweats or palpitations; get senior help.

ACUTE ASTHMA

Clues: SOB, wheeze, PEF <50% of best**, RR >25/min, HR >110/min, cannot complete sentences in 1 breath.

- Attach sats monitor.
- 40–60% O_2 through high-flow mask, e.g. Hudson mask.
- Salbutamol 5 mg neb in O_2: repeat up to every 15 min if life threatening.

- Ipratropium 0.5 mg neb in O_2: repeat up to every 4 h if life threatening or fails to respond to salbutamol,
- Prednisolone 40 mg po od for at least 5 days. Hydrocortisone 100 mg qds iv can be given if unable to swallow or retain tablets.

Both prednisolone and hydrocortisone can be given if very ill.

> **Life-threatening features**
> - PEF <33% of best**.
> - O_2 sats <92%.
> - PaO_2 <8.0 kPa, $PaCO_2$ >4.6 kPa or pH <7.35.
> - Silent chest, cyanosis or ↓respiratory effort.
> - ↓HR, ↓BP or dysrhythmia.
> - Exhaustion, confusion or coma.
> **Or predicted best (see p. 153/4).

If life-threatening features (☠NB: patient may not always *appear* distressed ☠); get senior help and consider the following:

- *$MgSO_4$ ivi*: 8 mmol over 20 min (= 2 g – 4 ml of 50% solution).
- *Aminophylline iv*: attach cardiac monitor and give loading dose* of 5 mg/kg iv over 20 min then ivi at 0.5–0.7 mg/kg/h.
  ☠**If already taking maintenance po aminophylline/ theophylline, omit loading dose* and check levels ASAP to guide dosing.**☠
- *iv salbutamol*: 5 µg/min initially (then up to 20 µg/min according to response): back-to-back or continuous nebs now often preferred.
- Call anaesthetist for consideration of ITU care or intubation. Initiate this during the above steps if deteriorating.

COPD EXACERBATION

Clues: SOB, wheeze, RR >25/min, HR >110.

- *Attach sats monitor* and do baseline ABGs.
- *28% O_2 via Venturi mask*; should be *prescribed on drug chart*. ↑dose cautiously if hypoxia continues, but repeat ABGs to ensure CO_2 not ↑ing and (more importantly) pH not ↓ing.

- *Ipratropium 0.5 mg neb* in O_2: repeat up to every 4 h if very ill.
- *Salbutamol 5 mg neb* in O_2: repeat up to every 15 min if very ill (seldom necessary >hourly).
- *Prednisolone 30 mg po* then od for ≤2 wks (often 7–10 days). Some give 1st dose as hydrocortisone 200 mg iv – rarely used now unless unable to swallow.
- *Antibiotics* (see pp. 140–3) if 2 out of 3 of Hx of ↑ing SOB, ↑ing volume or ↑ing purulence of sputum.

If no improvement, consider:

- *Aminophylline ivi:* see management of asthma (p. 201) for details.
- Assisted ventilation: CPAP if just ↓PaO_2 or NIV (BIPAP) if also ↑$PaCO_2$; consider doxapram if NIV not available.
- Intubation: discuss with ITU/anaesthetist.

PULMONARY EMBOLISM

Clues: unlikely unless RR >20 and PaO_2 <10.7 kPa (or ↓O_2 sats).

- *60–100% O_2* if hypoxic. Care if COPD.
- *Analgesia:* if xs pain or distress, try paracetamol/ibuprofen first; consider opiates if severe or no response (☠ can ⇒ respiratory depression ☠).
- *Anticoagulation:* LMWH, e.g. dalteparin or enoxaparin. Once PE confirmed, load with warfarin (see pp. 171–3). Consider iv heparin if surgery being contemplated, or rapid reversal may be required*.

If massive PE, worsening hypoxia or cardiovascular instability (↓BP, RV strain/failure), seek senior help and consider:

- *Fluids ± inotropes:* if systolic BP <90 mmHg.
- *Thrombolysis (e.g. alteplase):* if ↓BP ± collapse.
- *Embolectomy*:* seek urgent cardiothoracic opinion.

EPILEPSY

Status epilepticus = seizures for >30 min **or** >1 episode without full
recovery in between. NB: >80% of epileptic seizures last <2 min;
if >5 min ⇒ ↑risk of developing into status epilepticus and need
prompt treatment.

NB: non-convulsive/absence seizures are missed easily. Keep in
mind non-epileptic (= "pseudo") seizures, esp if atypical fits.

- *Protect airway:* get senior help early if concerned.
- *Attach O_2 sats monitor* and *place in recovery position.*
- 60–100% O_2 (beware COPD).
- *Exclude or treat reversible metabolic causes:* esp ↓O_2, ↓glucose,
  ↓thiamine (esp in alcoholics), ↓pyridoxine (if child – esp
  neonate).
- *Diazepam 10 mg iv* over 2 min, preferable as Diazemuls
  (↓s thrombophlebitis), repeating if necessary at 5 mg/min to
  maximum of 20 mg. If no iv access, give 30 mg pr (or consider
  midazolam 5–10 mg im).
  ☠ Beware of respiratory depression; have flumazenil at hand. ☠
- *Check BP:* maintain or ↑mean arterial blood pressure to provide
  appropriate cerebral perfusion pressure: get senior help if
  concerned.

If no response get senior help and give:

- *Lorazepam ivi:* 0.1 mg/kg at 2 mg/min (can use lower rate
  of infusion). If not available on ward, give diazepam ivi:
  100 mg in 500 ml 5% glucose at 40 ml/h.

If no response after 10 min, call for anaesthetist and give:

- *Phenytoin iv:* see pp. 105–6 for dose. Monitor BP and HR
  (both can drop) and ECG (esp QTc, as arrhythmias not
  uncommon). Phenobarbital 10–15 mg/kg iv at 100 mg/min
  is an alternative.

If the above measures do not terminate seizures, refractory status epilepticus is present. Requires general anaesthesia with propofol or thiopental in a specialised unit.

DKA

Clues: ketotic breath, Kussmaul's (deep/rapid) breathing, dehydration, confusion/↓GCS.

- *Initial measures:* O_2 if hypoxic, insert NGT if coma, weigh patient (if possible). Consider central line (esp if ↓↓pH or Hx of HF), but urinary catheter often sufficient (insert if no urine after 2–3 h).
- *iv fluids:* initially 0.9% saline according to individual patient needs (guided by urine output ± CVP). The following is a guide:
  - *If severe dehydration,* i.e. shock, oliguria or ARF (in this context = urea >21 mmol/l or creatinine >350 mmol/l), give 1st litre over 30 min, 2nd litre over 1 h and 3rd litre over 2 h. Consider colloid if ↓↓BP or no improvement in hydration.
  - *Otherwise* give more slowly, e.g. 2 l over 4 h, then 1 l over 4 h.
  - Add KCl once K^+ <5.5 mmol/l, as can ↓rapidly dt insulin (but do not give KCl in 1st litre unless K^+ <3.5 mmol/l). Roughly 20–30 mmol needed per litre during rehydration: adjust to individual response with regular checks (easiest and quickest done with ABG machines: most give K^+ levels, and ABGs also needed regularly for pH monitoring; can also use venous samples as long as put in ABG or other heparinised syringe).
- *Insulin:* as soluble insulin ivi (e.g. Actrapid). A sensible start is 6 units/h, ↑ing to 12 units/h if no ↓BG w/in 2 h. Higher doses can ⇒ too rapid a fall in BG and K^+ (aim for ↓BG of 3–6 mmol/h). If no ivi facilities available, give 10 units iv stat (↓dose if BG <20). Once BG <12, change iv fluids to 5% glucose and start insulin sliding scale (see p. 167), adjusting to response but ideally maintaining min rate of 4 units/h with sufficient glucose ivi (if insulin continued, speed of ketone clearance ↑s; if BG <5, do not stop insulin but ↑rate of glucose ivi or switch to 10% solution). Continue until ketones cleared (check urine ± blood),

pH normal and eating/drinking; then switch to sc regimen
(see p. 169 for advice).

- *Heparin:* if comatose or hyperosmolar (>350 mosmol/l), give
  LMWH (or unfractionated heparin 5000 units sc bd/tds).
  Continue until mobile.

Consider:

- *Antibiotics:* search for and treat infection. NB: rely on CRP more
  than WCC (WCC can be artificially ↑d) and temperature can be
  normal even in severe infections ∴ dipstick urine and send urine,
  blood and any other relevant cultures (consider CXR). If suspect
  infection and no clear cause, start blind Rx, e.g. cefotaxime 1 g
  bd iv (or other 3rd-generation cephalosporin).
- *Bicarbonate:* if severe acidosis (e.g. pH <7); very rarely needed
  and potentially dangerous. Get senior help if concerned.
- *HDU/ITU:* for one-to-one nursing ± ventilation if required.

Watch for complications: *electrolyte Δs* (esp ↓Na^+, ↓K^+, ↓Mg^{++},
↓PO_4), TE (esp DVT/PE), *cerebral oedema* (↓GCS, papilloedema,
false-localising cranial nerve palsies), *infections* (esp aspiration
pneumonia).

HONK

Clues: as for DKA, but no ketones, normal pH, ↑glucose,
↑dehydration and ↑confusion. Generally ↑age of patient and ↑length
of Hx of decline (NB: may be 1st presentation and no past Hx).
Can also be precipitated by steroids and thiazides.

- *Initial measures:* as DKA; see p. 204.
- *iv fluids:* as DKA, but can correct dehydration more slowly
  (will have occurred more slowly and also ↓s risk of electrolyte
  abnormalities). A rough guide is 1 l of 0.9% saline over 1 h, then
  2 l over 4 h ×2, then 1 l over 4 h. Less KCl will be needed, as less
  insulin will be used. NB: can remain in circulatory collapse
  despite clinically adequate fluid replacement; if so, give 500 ml

colloid and monitor CVP. Consider 0.45% saline if Na^+
>155 mmol/l; get senior (ideally specialist) help first.
- *Insulin:* start at lower dose than DKA (e.g. 2 units/h ivi).
  Again aim to ↓BG by 3–6 mmol/h and continue ivi for ⩾24 h
  (adding glucose if necessary to keep BG normal) before switching
  to sc regimen.
- *Heparin:* iv or LMWH (see pp. 174–7). Always give, as
  ↑↑osmolality ⇒ ↑risk of TE (and consider TEDS).

Consider:

- *Antibiotics:* search for and treat infection, as above.

Watch for complications, esp TE (CVA, IHD) and ARF.

↓GLUCOSE

Treat if <2.5 mmol/l or symptoms: ↑sympathetic drive (↑HR,
sweating, aggression/behavioural Δs), seizures or confusion/↓GCS.

- *Glucose orally:* esp sugary drinks or mouth gel (e.g. Hypostop).
  Miss this step if severe, but can be useful if delays in iv access.
- *Glucose 20–50 ml of 50%* iv stat via large Venflon. Always flush
  liberally with saline as 50% glucose is very viscous and will act
  slowly otherwise. Repeat if necessary. A brisk 5–20% glucose ivi
  can be used if only mild symptoms or until 50% glucose found,
  but beware of fluid overload if HF.
- *Glucagon 1 mg* im/iv stat: if very low glucose or no iv access.

NB: think of and correct any causes, esp xs DM Rx, alcohol
withdrawal, liver failure, aspirin OD (rarely Addison's disease, ↓T4).

THYROTOXIC CRISIS

Clues: ↑HR/AF, fever, abdominal pain, D&V, tremor, agitation,
confusion, coma. Look for goitre, Grave's eye disease.

- O_2: if hypoxic.
- *0.9% saline ivi:* slowly as per individual needs (care if HF).

- *Propranolol 40 mg tds po:* aim for HR <100 and titrate up dose if necessary (if β-blocker CI, give diltiazem 60–120 mg qds po). If ↑↑HR, give propranolol iv 1 mg over 1 min, repeating if necessary every 2 min to max total of 10 mg.
- *Digoxin and LMWH* (if AF): DC shock rarely works until euthyroid ∴ load with 500 μg iv over 30 min then 250 μg iv over 30 min every 2 h until HR <100 (up to max total of 1.5 mg).
- *Carbimazole:* 15–30 mg qds po (↓ later under specialist advice).
- *Lugol's solution (iodine):* 0.1–0.3 ml tds po (normally for 1 wk). Start 4 h after carbimazole.
- *Hydrocortisone:* 100 mg qds iv (or dexamethasone 4 mg qds po).

Consider:

- *Treat any heart failure* (common if fast AF), e.g. furosemide.
- *Antibiotics:* if evidence/suspicion of infection, e.g. 3rd-generation cephalosporin iv, such as cefotaxime 1 g bd iv.
- *Cooling measures:* paracetamol, sponging.

If vomiting, insert NGT to avoid aspiration and for drug administration.

MYXOEDEMA COMA

Clues: 'facies', goitre, thyroidectomy scar, ↓temperature, ↓HR, ↓reflexes, ↓glucose, seizures, coma. NB: Ψ features common.

- O_2: if hypoxic.
- *Glucose iv:* if hypoglycaemic (often coexists); see p. 206.
- *0.9% saline ivi:* slowly as per individual needs (care if HF).
- *Liothyronine* (= T_3 = tri-iodothyronine): 5–20 μg ivi bd for ⩾2 days then ↑dose gradually with endocrinologist's advice before converting to thyroxine po. Liothyronine can precipitate angina; slow down ivi if occurs.
- *Hydrocortisone:* 100 mg iv tds, esp if suspect hypopituitarism (much more likely if no goitre or past Hx of Rx for ↑T_4).

Consider:

- *Rewarming measures:* e.g. Bair-Hugger, warm iv fluids (and O_2).
- *Antibiotics:* infections are common and may have precipitated decline ∴ have low threshold for aggressive Rx (e.g. iv 3rd-generation cephalosporin).
- *Ventilation/ITU:* condition has high mortality.

ADDISONIAN CRISIS

Clues: ↓BP, ↑HR, ↓glucose, ↑K^+/↓Na^+, Hx of chronic high-dose steroid Rx with missed doses or intercurrent illness*?

- O_2 if cyanosed.
- *Glucose iv:* if hypoglycaemic; see p. 206.
- *Steroids:* usually hydrocortisone 100 mg iv stat then qds (ensure blood sample for cortisol and ACTH taken before first dose if Dx is not certain). Give 1st dose as dexamethasone 8 mg iv if Synacthen test planned (hydrocortisone affects test results). Consider fludrocortisone once stable.
- *Fluids iv:* colloid ± central line if ↓↓BP.
- *Antibiotics:* look for and treat infection*: dipstick urine, MSU, CXR and blood cultures. If in doubt, start Rx (e.g. iv 3rd-generation cephalosporin such as cefotaxime 1 g bd iv).

ELECTROLYTE DISTURBANCES

↑K^+

K^+ >6 mmol/l considered dangerous. *Is haemolysis of sample possible cause?* Ring lab ± repeat sample if suspicious.

If K^+ >6.5 mmol/l or ECG Δs (tall tented T waves, QRS >0.12 s (>3 small squares), loss of P waves or sinusoidal pattern) the following is needed:

- *Attach cardiac monitor* (+ECG if possible): risk of arrhythmias.
- *10 ml of 10% Ca^{2+} gluconate iv* over 2 min for cardioprotection, or 10 ml of 10% CaCl iv at ≤1 ml/min (often found in crash trolleys).

- *10 units insulin* (e.g. Actrapid) + 50 ml 50% glucose ivi over 30 min: stimulates cellular membrane H^+/K^+ pumps $\therefore \downarrow$s plasma K^+ levels. Beware of too rapid a drop as this may precipitate arrhythmias: aim for drop of 1–2 mmol/l over 30–60 min.
- Consider *salbutamol 5–20 mg nebs:* utilises K^+-lowering fx.

For all patients with $\uparrow K^+$:

- *Look for and treat causes*, esp ARF (consider dialysis) and drugs; e.g. iv KCl, oral K^+ supplements, ACE-i, ARBs, K^+-sparing diuretics, NSAIDs. Also ciclosporin but don't adjust without specialist advice.

If $\uparrow K^+$ persists:

- Calcium Resonium 15 g tds/qds po; takes $\geq$24 h to work.

$\downarrow K^+$

<2.5 mmol/l $\Rightarrow$ risk of arrhythmias: attach cardiac monitor.

- *1 l normal saline (0.9%) + 40 mmol KCl* over 4 h. If unstable or arrhythmias develop, seek senior help. KCl can be given quicker but non-specialist wards may not allow >10 mmol/h and patient may not tolerate fast peripheral ivi due to pain (consider central line).
- *Oral K^+ replacement* should also be commenced (e.g. Sando-K, Slow-K 2 tablets tds, or as much as can be tolerated – unpleasant taste!). Beware of overshooting later, esp if cause removed.

NB: po replacement is often sufficient if K^+ >2.5 mmol/l and no clinical features/ECG Δs (small T waves or large U waves).

$\uparrow Ca^{2+}$

>2.65 mmol/l is abnormal. Symptoms usually start once >2.9 mmol/l. *Clues:* bones (pain, esp consider metastases), stones (renal colic $\pm$ ARF), groans (abdominal pains, constipation $\pm$ vomiting; polyuria and thirst common) and psychic moans (inc confusion).

If >3.5 mmol/l or severe symptoms treat urgently as follows:

- 0.9% *saline ivi*: average requirements 4–6 l over 24 h
  (↓ if elderly/HF). Monitor fluid balance carefully and correct
  electrolytes.

If insufficient improvement in Ca^{2+} levels or symptoms get senior
help and consider:

- *Loop diuretic* (e.g. furosemide): consider once rehydrated.
- *Bisphosphonate* (e.g. pamidronate) esp if ↑PTH or malignancy.
- *Calcitonin*: if no response to bisphosphonate.
- *Steroids*: if sarcoid, lymphoma, myeloma or vitamin D toxicity.
- *Dialysis*: if ARF or life-threatening symptoms.

OVERDOSES

Unless you are familiar with the up-to-date Mx of the specific
overdose in question, the following sources should always be
consulted:

- *Toxbase website (www.spib.axl.co.uk)*: authoritative and
  updated regularly. Should be used in the 1st instance to check
  clinical features and Mx of the poison(s) in question. You will
  need to sign in under your departmental account; if your
  department is not registered, contact your A&E department to
  obtain a username and password.
- *National Poisons Information Service (NPIS)*: if in UK phone
  0870 600 6266 (if in Ireland 01 809 2526) for advice if unsure
  of Toxbase instructions and for rarer/mixed overdoses.

GENERAL MEASURES

- *GI decontamination*: activated charcoal (and, rarely, gastric
  lavage) can be given if w/in 1 h* of significant OD ingestion.
  Both are CI if ↓GCS (unless ET tube in situ). Gastric lavage is
  also CI if corrosive OD or risk of GI haemorrhage/perforation.

Activated charcoal can be repeated with certain drugs but does not work with others (most notably, lithium, iron, organophosphates, ethylene glycol, ethanol, methanol). Consult Toxbase ± NPIS for severe or unusual poisoning, as routine GI decontamination is no longer recommended.

- Check paracetamol and aspirin levels in all patients who are unable to give an accurate Hx of the exact poisons ingested.

*Unless drug is MR preparation or causes delayed gastric emptying (e.g. salicylates, opiates, TCAs, theophyllines, sympathomimetics). In such cases, GI decontamination can be given later; exactly how much longer is a controversial issue, so contact NPIS if you are concerned about a potentially serious ingestion. See Toxbase for dosage guide for activated charcoal.

PARACETAMOL

Significant OD = ingestion of 150 mg/kg or 12 g (whichever is smaller). If risk factors (see below), 75 mg/kg should be used instead. NB: if patient weighs >110 kg, use 110 kg (rather than their actual weight) for these calculations.

> **Risk factors in paracetamol OD**
> - Taking enzyme-inducing drugs, e.g. carbamazepine, pheno-barbital, primidone, phenytoin, rifampicin, St John's wort.
> - Regularly consumes alcohol in xs of recommended amounts.
> - Malnourished and likely to be glutathione-depletc, e.g. anorexia, alcoholism, cystic fibrosis, HIV infection.

Initial management

This depends on time since ingestion.

0–8 h post-ingestion:

- *Activated charcoal:* if w/in 1 h of significant OD.
- *Acetylcysteine:* wait until 4 h post-ingestion before taking urgent sample for paracetamol levels (results are meaningless until this time). If presents at 4–8 h post-ingestion, take sample ASAP.

If levels above the treatment line (see below), give the following acetylcysteine regimen:

- *Initially* 150 mg/kg in 200 ml 5% glucose ivi over 15 min.
- *Then* 50 mg/kg in 500 ml 5% glucose ivi over 4 h.
- *Then* 100 mg/kg in 1000 ml 5% glucose ivi over 16 h.

> Do not delay acetylcysteine beyond 8 h post-ingestion if waiting
> for paracetamol levels result and significant OD (beyond 8 h,
> efficacy ↓s substantially) – ivi can be stopped if levels come back
> as below treatment line and INR, ALT and creatinine normal.

8–15 h post-ingestion:

- *Acetylcysteine:* give above regimen ASAP if significant OD taken.
  Do not wait for urgent paracetamol level result. Acetylcysteine
  can be stopped if level later turns out to be below treatment line
  and timing of the OD is certain **and** patient asymptomatic with
  normal INR, creatinine and ALT.

15–24 h post-ingestion:

- *Acetylcysteine:* give above regimen ASAP unless certain that
  significant OD has not been taken. Do not wait for paracetamol
  level result. Presenting this late ⇒ severe risk, and treatment lines
  are unreliable: always finish course of acetylcysteine.

>24 h post-ingestion:

- Acetylcysteine is controversial when presenting this late. Monitor
  as below and discuss the individual case with NPIS.

NB: use high-risk line if any of the risk factors on p. 211 apply.

> *Important points regarding acetylcysteine*
> - Have lower threshold for initiating Rx if doubts over timing
>   of OD, if ingestion was staggered, if presents 24–36 h
>   post-ingestion, or if evidence of LF/severe toxicity regardless
>   of time since ingestion. Contact NPIS if unsure.

(Continued on p. 214)

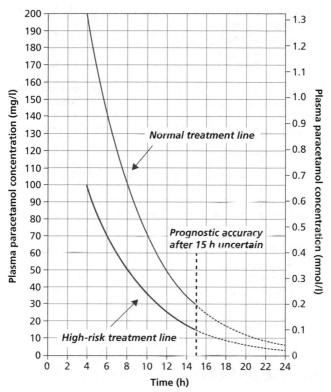

Figure 11 Treatment lines for acetylcysteine treatment of paracetamol overdose.
Reproduced courtesy of Alun Hutchings and University of Wales College of Medicine
Therapeutics and Toxicology Centre.

- Anaphylactoid reactions common esp at initial faster rates. If occurs stop ivi and most cases will resolve. Give antihistamine (e.g. chlorphenamine 10–20 mg iv over 1 min) if required. Consider corticosteroids only if reaction severe and give salbutamol nebs if significant bronchospasm. Once reaction settles restart acetylcysteine ivi at 50 mg/kg over 4 h. Past Hx of such reactions is not an absolute CI to future treatment; **either** pretreat with chlorphenamine 10 mg iv and ensure 1st ivi not given too quickly **or** give 1st ivi at slower rate (over 1 h rather than 15 min) but latter of these 2 options is unlicensed.
- Can ⇒ mildly ↑INR itself; ∴ if after treatment ALT is normal but INR is ≤1.3 no further monitoring or treatment is needed. But if ALT is ↑, continue acetylcysteine ivi at rate of 150 mg/kg given over 24 h (unless 2nd overdose taken no loading dose needed).

Subsequent management

GCS and urine output should be monitored closely. Patients should be *medically* fit for discharge once acetylcysteine ivi is completed, and INR, ALT, creatinine and HCO_3^- ($\pm$pH) subsequently checked to be normal and stable (*psychiatric* clearance for discharge may take longer).

If acetylcysteine not given w/in 8 h of OD, inpatient observation for 3–4 days recommended to check liver and renal function (INR and creatinine are best parameters respectively).

If abnormalities detected, consult Toxbase ± NPIS for consideration of further acetylcysteine and specialist referral. On discharge, advise all patients to return to hospital if abdominal pains or vomiting develop.

ASPIRIN

- *Consider activated charcoal ± gastric lavage*: if w/in 1 h of OD of >120 mg/kg. Aspirin delays gastric emptying (esp if enteric-coated tablets), ∴ both can be considered >1 h after ingestion and activated charcoal can be repeated later if salicylate levels continue to rise despite measures below; contact NPIS for advice.

- *Monitor* U&Es, glucose, clotting, ABGs (or venous pH and HCO_3^-) and fluid balance (often need large volumes of iv fluid). Salicylate levels needed if OD of >120 mg/kg; take sample at least 2 h post-ingestion if symptomatic or 4 h post-ingestion if not symptomatic, repeating in both cases 2 h later if severe toxicity suspected in case of delayed absorption (repeating until levels↓).

If abnormalities detected, get senior help or contact ITU for specialist advice, and then consider the following:

- *Sodium bicarbonate:* 1.5 l of 1.26% iv over 2 h (or 225 ml of 8.4%). Give only if metabolic acidosis, salicylate levels >500 mg/l (3.6 mmol/l) and serum K^+ levels either normal or have been corrected. Ensure given through patent cannula (risk of tissue necrosis if extravasation). Such alkalinisation of urine can itself ↓K^+ so iv KCl replacement may be needed; monitor K^+ closely. Consider further 225 ml ivi of 8.4% sodium bicarbonate to keep urine pH at 7.5–8.5. Remeasure salicylate levels to check Rx has been effective.
- *Haemodialysis:* if salicylate levels >700 mg/l (5.1 mmol/l) or unresponsive to the above measures. Also consider if ARF, CCF, non-cardiac pulmonary oedema, severe metabolic acidosis, convulsions or any CNS fx that are not resolved by correction of pH. Have lower threshold if age >70 years.

OPIATES

Clues: pinpoint pupils, ↓respiratory rate, ↓GCS, drug chart and Hx/signs of opiate abuse (e.g. track marks).

- O_2 + maintain airway ± ventilatory support.
- *Naloxone* 0.4–2.0 mg iv (or im) stat initially, repeating after 2 min if no response. See p. 97 for subsequent dosing.

BENZODIAZEPINES

- O_2 + maintain airway ± ventilatory support.
- Consider *flumazenil:* see p. 61 for dosage.

> *Flumazenil is not recommended as a diagnostic test and should not be given routinely.* Risk of inducing fits (esp if epileptic), withdrawal syndrome (if habituated to benzodiazepines) or arrhythmias (esp if coingested TCA or amphetamine-like drug of abuse). If in any doubt, get senior opinion and never give without normal ECG and excluding patient habituation to benzodiazepines, unless 'in extremis' and benzodiazepines are clearly the cause.

COMA

Glasgow Coma Scale (GCS): standardised assessment of coma.

Motor response	Verbal response	Eye opening
6 Obeys commands	5 Orientated	4 Spontaneous
5 Localises pain	4 Confused	3 Responds to speech
4 Withdraws to pain	3 Inappropriate	2 Responds to pain
3 Flexes to pain	2 Incomprehensible	1 None
2 Extends to pain	1 None	
1 No response to pain		

GCS 13–15 = minor injury
GCS 9–12 = moderate injury
GCS <9   = severe injury

NB: drops of ≥2 are often significant.

To remember GCS use **MoVE** for 3 categories and mnemonic **'OLDFEZ OCEAN SOON'**, visualising an old fez (Moroccan hat) floating down a river that will soon arrive at the ocean!
Motor: Obeys, Localises, Draws away, Flexor, Extensor, Zero.
Verbal: Orientated, Confused, Explicit (or eX rated), Absolute rubbish, None.
Eye: Spontaneous, Orders only, Ouch only, None.

> **Causes of ↓GCS = DIM TOPS**
> - *Drugs:* alcohol, insulin, sedatives, overdoses (esp opiates/benzos).
> - *Infections:* sepsis, meningitis, encephalitis.
> - *Metabolic:* ↑/↓glucose, ↓T_4, Addison's, renal/liver failure.
> - *Trauma Hx:* ?unwitnessed fall or extradural 'lucid interval'.
> - *O_2 deficiency:* any cause of ↓O_2 (NB: ↑CO_2 is also a cause).
> - *Perfusion:* CVA (inc SAH), MI, PE./*Pressure:* ↑ICP.
> - *Seizures:* post-ictal fx and non-convulsive status aren't obvious.

COGNITIVE IMPAIRMENT

1. **(A)MTS:** (Abbreviated) Mental Test Score – most basic assessment of cognition; popular with physicians due to brevity (esp for use on the elderly). <8/10 is abnormal (i.e. dementia and/or delirium).

W	World War II: what year did it end?[1]
H	Hospital (what is name of building are you in?).
A	Address: 42 West St (ask to repeat and remember*).
T	Time: to the nearest hour.
Y	Year.
E	Elizabeth II (who is current monarch?)[1]
A	Age (of patient).
R	Recognition of 2 persons: e.g. Dr and other[2].
B	Birthday (patient's date of birth).
C	Count backwards from 20 to 1.
?	? Can you remember the address*.

[1] If culturally inappropriate change to relevant question or omit.
[2] If alone with patient omit.
If questions omitted, record why and reduce denominator of score.

2. **MMSE:** Mini Mental State Examination; popular and best validated basic cognitive assessment. **Questions to ask are in bold.**
Orientation:
Time – (1–3) **Date?** 1 point for each for day, month and year.   5
(4) **Season?** (5) **Day of week?**

Place – (1) **Country?** (2) **County/state (or large city)?**   5
        (3) **Town (or city area)?** (4) **Building?** (5) **Floor?**

Registration: Say[1] **ball, flag, tree.** Repeat until success or   3
        5 attempts.

Attention/concentration: **Spell 'WORLD' backwards**[2].   5

Recall: **Can you remember those 3 items?** (ball, flag, tree).   3

3-stage command: **Take paper in R hand, fold in half and put**   3
        on floor

Language: **What is this?** Point to pen and then wristwatch.   2
        Repeat exactly after me: 'No ifs, ands or buts.'   1

Reading/comprehension: **Do what the sentence below instructs**[3].   1

Praxis: **Write a sentence of your choice.** Provide dotted line.   1
        Copy this shape as best you can alongside it[4].   1

1 Precede with 'I will mention 3 objects to you. Please repeat them
to me once I have finished all 3.' Allow 1 sec between objects. At
end say 'I will ask you to remember these later' which is tested in
Recall in next but one section – should be done after 1 min.
2 'Serial 7s' can also be used which obviously tests calculation too so
remember to take into account premorbid numeracy skills.
3 Write out in large, clear capital letters 'CLOSE YOUR EYES'.
4 Only correct if makes 4-sided shape formed by 2
        intersecting pentagons.

- Allow 1 min for tasks, except 30 sec for 3-stage command and
  writing of sentence.
- Score < 25/30 abnormal (i.e. dementia and/or delirium). 25–27
  is borderline. *NB: frontal lobe tests not covered; useful
  to add.*

COMMON LABORATORY REFERENCE VALUES

NB: normal ranges often vary between laboratories. The ranges
given here are deliberately narrow to minimise missing abnormal
results, but this means that your result may be normal for your
laboratory's range, which should always be checked if possible.

Biochemistry

Na$^+$	135–145 mmol/l
K$^+$	3.5–5.0 mmol/l
Urea	2.5–6.5 mmol/l
Creatinine	70–110 μmol/l
Ca^{2+}	2.15–2.65 mmol/l
PO$_4$	0.8–1.4 mmol/l
Albumin	35–50 g/l
Protein	60–80 g/l
Mg^{2+}	0.75–1.0 mmol/l
Cl$^-$	95–105 mmol/l
Glucose (fasting)	3.5–5.5 mmol/l
LDH	70–250 iu/l
CK	25–195* u/l (↑ in blacks)
Trop I	<0.4 ng/ml (= μg/l)
Trop T	<0.1 ng/ml (= μg/l)
D-dimers	<0.5** mg/l
Bilirubin	3–17 μmol/l
ALP	30–130 iu/l
AST	3–31 iu/l
ALT	3–35 iu/l
GGT	7–50* iu/l
Amylase	0–180 u/dl
Cholesterol	3.9–5.2 mmol/l
Triglycerides	0.5–1.9 mmol/l
Urate	0.2–0.45 mmol/l
CRP	0–10 mg/l

Haematology

Hb male	13.5–17.5 g/dl
Hb female	11.5–15.5 g/dl
Pt	150–400 × 10^9/l
WCC	4–11 × 10^9/l

*Sex differences exist: females occupy the lower end of the range.

**D-dimer normal range can vary with different test protocols: check with your lab!

Haematology (Continued)

NØ	$2.0–7.5 \times 10^9/l$ (40–75%)
LØ	$1.3–3.5 \times 10^9/l$ (20–45%)
EØ	$0.04–0.44 \times 10^9/l$ (1–6%)
PCV (= Hct)	0.37–0.54* l/l
MCV	76–96 fl
ESR	<age in years *(+10 in women)*/2
HbA$_{1C}$	2.3–6.5%

Clotting

APTT	35–45 s
APTT ratio	0.8–1.2
INR	0.8–1.2

Haematinics

Iron	11–30 μmol/l
Transferrin	2–4 g/l
TIBC	45–72 μmol/l
Serum folate	1.8–11 μg/l
B$_{12}$	200–760 pg/ml (= ng/l)

Arterial blood gases

PaO$_2$	>10.6 kPa
PaCO$_2$	4.7–6.0 kPa
pH	7.35–7.45
HCO$_3^-$	24–30 mmol/l
Base xs	± 2 mmol/l

Thyroid function

Thyroxine (total T$_4$)	70–140 nmol/l
Thyroxine (free T$_4$)	9–22 pmol/l
TSH	0.5–5 mU/l

*Sex differences exist: females occupy the lower end of the range.

INDEX